LET'S GET STEPPIN!

Saving the Next Generation...

Pedometer Walking

LET'S GET STEPPIN!

Saving the Next Generation...

Pedometer Walking

By

Billie Jean King

"Let's Get Steppin! Saving the Next Generation…Pedometer Walking

Copyright©2011 by: Billie Jean King

ISBN# 978-0-615-33268-0

Published by: BJK Publications

Printed in the United States

Cover Design: by.Tywebbin Creations

Interior Photos: Shutter Stock

For further inquires or information:
www.billiejeankingatlast.com
letsgetsteppin11@aol.com

Dedication

*I dedicate this book to my daughter, Shari Amour King-Ignont
For realizing the necessity to alternative food choices.*

<u>*My sister:*</u>

*Millie Lee Abram, for your sacrificial efforts
during your rehabilitation process.*

<u>*My aunt:*</u>
*Elnora Dumas, for your courageous and submissive
attitude demonstrated during the transitional process
of leaving your home.*

<u>*My aunt:*</u>
*Dorothy Stokes, may you be comforted, in your lengthy
battle with Alzheimer's*

&

*My brothers, James, Henry and A.C. and my entire family in Louisiana who is battling with obesity and the
associated complications.*

Table of Contents:

INTRODUCTION

Since this is the introduction, let me tell you a little about me. My name is Billie Jean King. This is my second book. My first published book is a fictional love story novel entitled, *"At Last."* After seeing the back cover, you know that I'm not the world renowned tennis player of all times, **Billie Jean King.** I think now would be a good time for me to thank her for all of the warm receptions that I've received while sharing her name, and to answer the question that I've been asked a zillion times. *"How did you get her name?"* It's kind of obvious…but, there's a little story behind it.

A fan since high school; I would storm to the locker room to dress for P.E., hoping to be the first on the tennis court to secure a racket. Not just any racket, there was only one that bore the name of **Billie Jean King**. During my entire sales career of over twenty years, many doors and receptive phone calls were always welcomed at the mere mention of her name. More than often it aided in turning a cold call into a warm one, whether by phone or in person.

In the early seventies when she resided in Emeryville, I received a letter intended for her requesting her presence at a speaking engagement. With regrets, I returned it to the sender of course; I desired to keep it as a show off souvenir. After that, I couldn't resist the notion to think, *"Wow… what if I'd received one of her checks?"* Hey…it was just my imagination.

Acquiring her name, well… fortunately, it was an oops! You see, I was named another six letter name beginning with the letter "B". I dislike the name, so I'll refrain from mentioning it as not to offend anyone. Born in Louisiana, when my doctor filled out my birth certificate, he wrote, **Billie Jean** instead. Thank you! Thank you! Dr. Desoto. I guess mistakes can turn into a *good thing.* I'm proud to say that sharing your name has been sheer delight. It's been thirty plus years since you crushed Bobby Riggs; but whenever my I.D. is presented, or my name given, it still presents an opportunity to discuss that day, or the mere fascination that I share your name. Oftentimes people will voice, *"I bet you get tired of hearing that, ha?"* With a smile, I respond, **"No!" Thanks! Billie Jean.**

The premise of my book is to bring awareness to the effectiveness of the *pedometer* to a number of people who have yet to [experience] and realize its usefulness in tracking and monitoring their daily activity levels. I want to inspire and encourage everyday Americans like me who battle daily to ward off obesity and the associated complications of *hypertension, type II diabetics, high cholesterol levels, potential strokes and heart attacks.*

More than often books of testimonials are written after the *triumph*, but rarely during the *struggle*, whether it's grief [after] a death, illness, addiction, relationship break-up, and or weight loss. Managing my weight has been and I'm convinced that it will continue to be a lifetime concern, as I am certain that it will continue to be an issue for many Americans.

Although I've worn a pedometer for the past six years, the inspiration to put it to pen came over four years ago. In the summer of 2007, I'd watched Shaquille O'Neal's "Big Challenge" episode showing his hands on efforts to fight the war on obesity with our kids. In 2008 my granddaughter's weight became a note worthy concern. In engaging accounts, I will share in detail from an observational point of view, the psychological effects and the actual results that were achieved during the trial period of her wearing the pedometer.

Initially my goal was to share only the efficiency of the pedometer relative to kids. As circumstances of life unfolded for me; and hearing on the evening news daily the devastating effects of obesity; I felt led to appeal to the adults as well. The more I contemplated the idea, the more sense that it made. Since my focus was kids, I realized that change had to begin in the mind and hearts of the parent before any implementation of change could occur for a child. Like most behaviors, whether it's inherited, environmental, or learned; it can generally be traced back to the parent, which brings me to my next area of focus.

Consistent with so many families across the U.S., my family is plagued by history repeating itself in the form of obesity, or more commonly defined as a *generational curse*. My mission is to break the cycle of Obesity and the related diseases in my generation and the next generation of family members. I will share with you, [not advise], of the various changes that I've put into practice to ensure me of the opportunity for a healthier life style than my parents and grandparents.

My research discovered six to eight books in print on promoting the use of the *pedometer* for monitoring activity levels and walking. I'm certain that there's more, however, these were sufficient in assisting me to draw my conclusions. Most were written by doctors or individuals directly related to the healthcare or fitness industry. Consequently, they all consisted of 200-300 plus pages of [good] and useful information on facts, causes, effects, diet and nutrition, relative to pedometer usage. The Information and recommended programs would prove beneficial to any potential reader. Traditionally, self help books of this nature generally speak to the mind of the reader.

I came away with the notion that a book needed to be written promoting the effectiveness of the pedometer to a *targeted segment of America*. It needed be relatable and **identifiable to readers such as *grandparents, big mama's, uncles, aunts, siblings and* cousins** who are battling daily with health complications resulting from a lack of movement and exercise.

It needed to be non-clinical, yet, promoting self awareness communicated through engaging story telling. Lastly, it needed to speak to the hearts of individuals as well as to the mind. It is said that a picture is worth a *thousand words*; I've incorporated colorful photos to aid in illustrating and supporting various topics.

More than a few times I tussled with the idea of holding off publishing this book until I'd attained my desired weight goal; I figured that it would be received or recognized as being a more effective or proven means, you know, *after the victory*. Then I was reminded that it's during the struggles of life is when encouragement, comfort, and strength is needed the most, whether you're the one that's receiving the support or giving it.

My aim is to be a contributing catalyst to help in bringing awareness and change to tackle the rising problem of Obesity in America. I've written this book in a practical and heartfelt manner. I believe that it will speak to and meet many of you in the exact place with you and your generation of family members. I've included charts that have tracked and monitored various careers, school kids and their extracurricular activates, all with the expressed purpose of stimulating consciousness to a simple little gadget; the *pedometer*, the next best thing since the "*stop watch*. I've created a blog to serve as a platform to [receive] or [provide] motivation, praise, share ideas or suggestions to those of us who have begun the journey, and to those who have yet to begin.

In chapter seven, in addition to discussing the need for a pedometer safety leash; I will also be introducing my line of *pedometer safety leashes* that were inspired by an actual need.

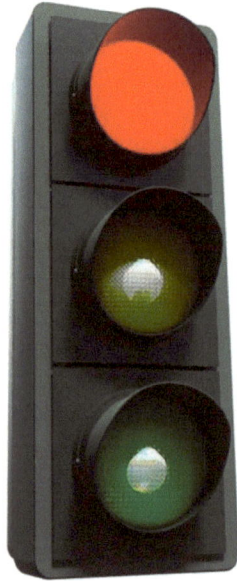

SAFETY NOTICE

Before embarking on any exercise regiment, diet, alternative foods, or suggestions relative to walking or physical fitness mentioned in this book, please consult with *a medical doctor*. The information compiled in this book was written from the prospective of a personal experience of the author. The author does not hold any credentials associated with health related issues.

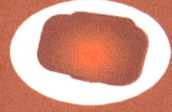

What is a Pedometer?

A Pedometer (pe-dom-eter) or step counter is a device in modern times usually portable and electronic or electromechanical that counts each step a person takes by detecting the motion of the person's hips. Because the distance of each person's step varies, an informal calibration performed by the user is required if a standardized distance (such as in kilometers or miles) is desired.

Who invented the pedometer?

Several people have been credited with inventing the pedometer, but the most likely inventor is Leonardo da Vinci. Others often mentioned as possible pedometer inventors are the English scientist Robert Hooke, Thomas Jefferson and the Romans of the third century.

Pedometer Usefulness:

There's nothing better than a good analogy to assist in identifying the significance of a matter that you're trying to convey or prove its value and worthiness. After careful deliberating; I settled on the "*stop watch*." Without the use of the *stop watch,* the sport of track and field would be limited to a group of fast runners with no means to track their speed, time, and distance. Imagine Jackie Joyner Kersey, or Maurice Green practicing without the use of a Trainer and a *stop watch*. Without it, there would be no effective method for the runner to determine and track their level of performance. It would be virtually impossible to set goals and advance to higher levels of running. The pedometer provides the exact incentive and functions to individuals who walk and need to monitor and set goals to increase their movement and activity levels.

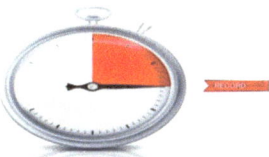

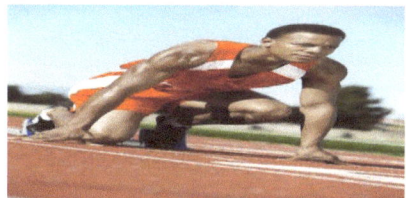

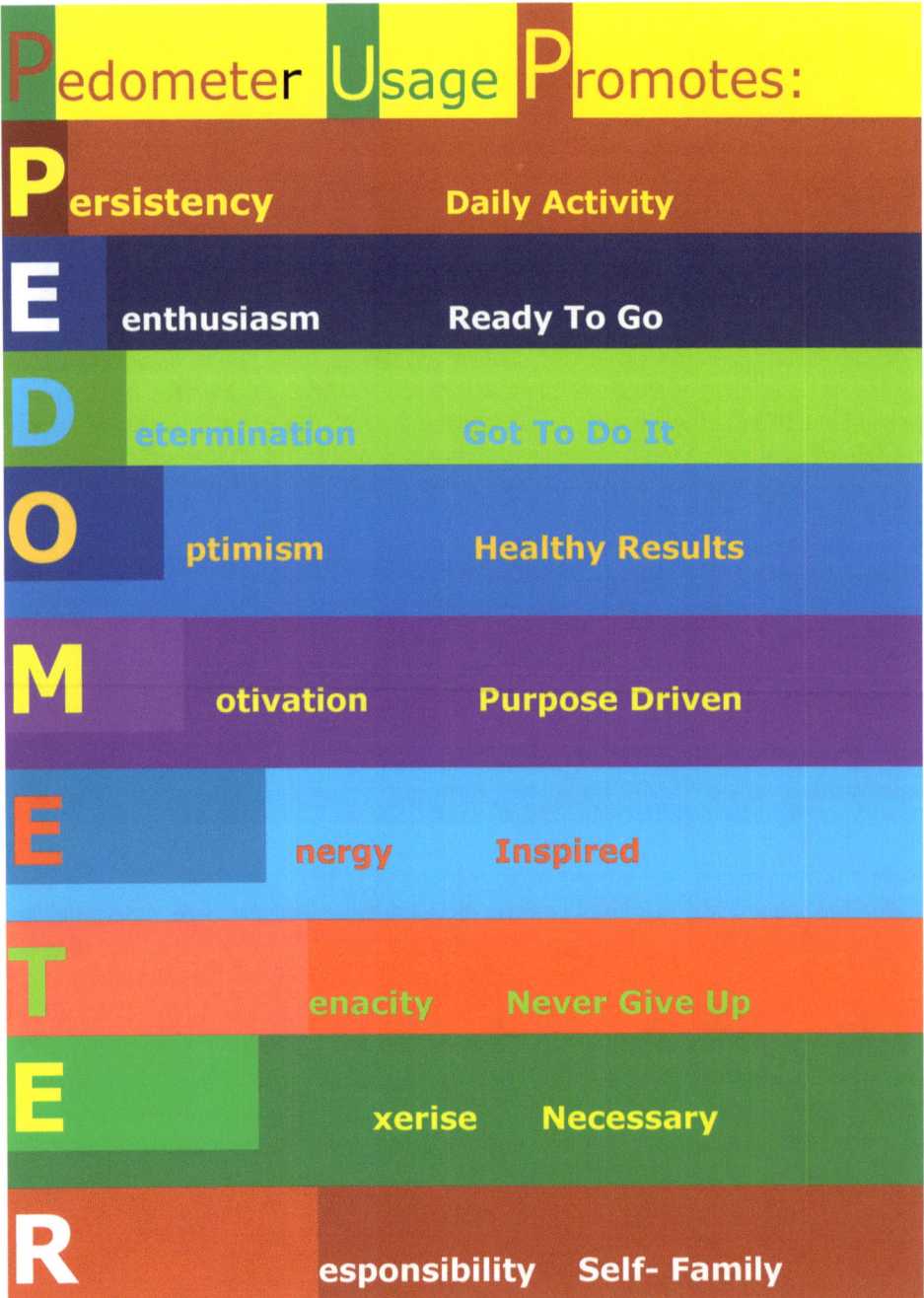

Pedometer Usage Promotes:

Persistency   Daily Activity

Enthusiasm   Ready To Go

Determination   Got To Do It

Optimism   Healthy Results

Motivation   Purpose Driven

Energy   Inspired

Tenacity   Never Give Up

Exerise   Necessary

Responsibility   Self- Family

Where do I wear my pedometer?

For maximum efficiency, it is recommended that the pedometer be worn on the waist, *in line with your knee.*

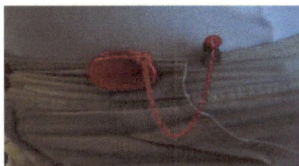

What If I am wearing a dress?

No problem! Depending on the size of your pedometer and the type of garment that you're wearing; the pedometer can be worn discreetly to your bra. Yeah, it works. You may have to do a little maneuvering to find the best spot, but it works. It works best when attached to the area where the bra and strap connect. (in the front of course.)

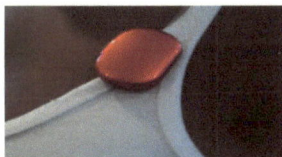

What Kind Should I Buy?

That's the million dollar question concerning pedometers. There are so—many pedometers on the market, and as much controversy as there are pedometers. I'm obviously *not qualified* to make any recommendations as to the accuracy of a particular type or brand of pedometer, and I'm going to refrain from disclosing the brand that I use. My goal is to provide you with enough information for you to make a conscious decision on the one that's affordable and works best for you, and your level of movement.

With anything that we purchase, price verses quality becomes a factor. Now, that's not always a bad thing. While compiling my data, I purchased two different brand of pedometers from Amazom.com costing $5.00 each, and another from a retailer costing $10.00, and mine, purchased from a pharmacy, costing $31.00. I tested all four taking 100 steps, and a one hour and fifteen minute walk. See the following chart for the results. Yes, I'm a slow walker.

Pedometer Price & Accuracy Face Off

Pedometer Cost	100 Step Count Test	1HR, Fifteen MIN. Goal 10K Steps
$5.00	77 Steps Counted	8600 Steps Counted
$5.00	105 Steps Counted	10,500 Steps Counted
$10.00	110 Steps Counted	10,350 Steps Counted
$31.00	103 Steps Counted	10,109 Steps Counted

You can see that the numbers are not significantly huge, except for one of the **$5.00** ones. Therefore, do not let the price be your determining factor. A large majority of individuals that I surveyed or interviewed that used the pedometer had received it as a free gift. Companies purchase them in bulk orders to give to their customers. HMO's and other healthcare organizations give them away at enrollment events and health fairs.

If you have one of those and the pedometer starts to register while holding it in your hand, as some have been reported, then you probably need to consider another one. I'm not implying that free pedometers will not get the job done. To ensure that the pedometer that you're going to use is in close proximity to your actual steps taken, take the 100-200 steps test. Start by walking and counting your steps while wearing the pedometer. If it's counting 10-200 steps off as in the chart above, don't sweat it. The goal is to get moving; you can always upgrade your pedometer later.

Remember, we're counting steps...*not heartbeats*. Try not to get side tracked by the inaccuracy of your pedometer compared to a friend, or reports from professionals and marketing companies suggesting that it needs to be this or that. There are so many variations of pedometers in the market place as well as online. Some have low and high level functionality modes. If you're technically challenged like me, you want to limit your pedometer functions. I've had several people to tell me that they became frustrated in their attempt to figure it out. If it requires extensive reading to get going, it probably has too many capabilities for you. Each morning I press one button and I'm good to go. Focusing too much on technicalities will hinder your agenda and render you discouraged.

Let's Get Steppin!

How accurate are our bathroom scales? We step on them every other morning to monitor our weight loss or gain, only to discover that we're 5 to 10 pounds over or under when we visit our doctor. And don't forget about the portable blood pressure monitor, again, it's never consistent with our physicians.

How accurate is your bathroom Scale...Blood Pressure Monitor?

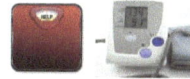

However, they do provide us with some level of monitoring to keep us on target and in a state of consciousness concerning our health. With that said; if you discover that your pedometer or your kids' pedometer is off as much as 1000k, and you've only walked 5000 steps, instead of 6000 steps...or 10,000 steps instead of 12,000 steps, *you are still a head of the game, and far better off when you were sitting on the couch watching TV.*

Any number of steps...is better than the alternative!

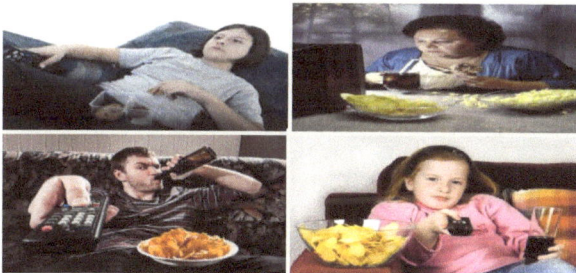

Although pedometers are common now, in earlier times they were used by runners to measure distances. In those times the pedometer was very important, especially to athletes. However, today they are mainly used for counting and recording the number of steps taken. The main reason for this is that walking has become a standard form of exercise and more strenuous activities are no longer required before someone is considered to be exercising.
Popular Article.Com by: Henry Calhoun, Oct.10, 2009

When Do I Wear My Pedometer?

If you're just beginning to walk using a pedometer, it's recommended that you wear it every day and all day until bedtime. Remember, the purpose of the pedometer is to track your steps and activity levels in the course of a day. Before you can begin setting goals, you need to know your current movement levels.

This will be interesting, if you're not a kid, then you'll behave as one. The anxiety to know the number of steps will get the best of you, that's part of the motivational aspect of using the pedometer. For one week, including weekends, track your daily routine by recording it on the data sheet provided in the back of the book. If you feel that you've adequately tracked a routine week, begin to set some realistic goals. *As always, consult with your physician before beginning your walking regiment.*

To get an accurate count of your daily activity levels, the monitoring should include your daily routine, e.g. work, play, school, sports, and exercise.

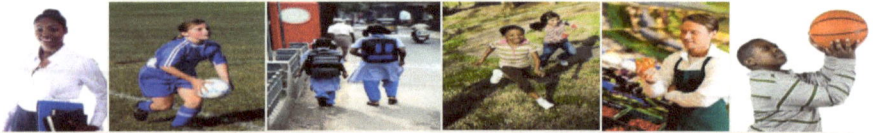

Benefits of Walking:

- Burns almost as many calories as jogging
- Eases back pains
- Slims your waist
- Lowers blood pressure
- Reduces levels of bad cholesterol
- Reduces heart attack risks
- Enhances Stamina & energy
- Lessons Anxiety & tension
- Improves muscle tone
- Easy on your joints
- Reduces appetite
- Increases aerobic capacity
- Slows down osteoporosis bone loss
- Can be done when you're traveling

(Reference: sportline.com)

Let's Get Steppin!

2

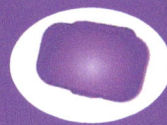

Obesity Awareness with Kids:

In the twenty first century, we have finally embraced the seriousness of Obesity with our youths. Thanks to our First Lady Michelle Obama's *"Let's Move Campaign"*, our educational system is being challenged to evaluate and implement changes in school lunch programs across the United States.

At a time when we're fighting to recover from the housing and financial crisis; America households suffers a third crisis, Obesity, and it's not limited to our kids. In light of the fact that we've been inundated with talk shows, the Surgeon General's report, magazine articles, health journals, all promoting healthy eating habits; yet, the problem seemingly continues to mount.

Healthcare experts recommend sixty plus minutes of daily physical activity for children to maintain optimum health. Some studies found that kids who exceed the recommended 12k steps needed for daily physical requirements and average up to 16k steps and above a day, are likely to maintain healthier weight levels.

To gain a better perspective on steps taken by different groups of people; the following study was taken by the (University of Arizona, Department of Consumer and family Sciences.)

- Children typically take **10,500 to 16000** steps per day (lower for girls than boy.)

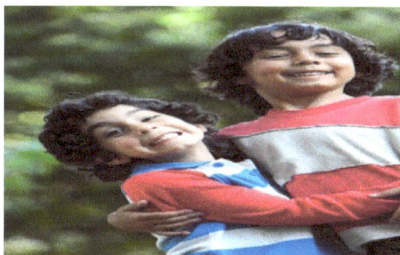

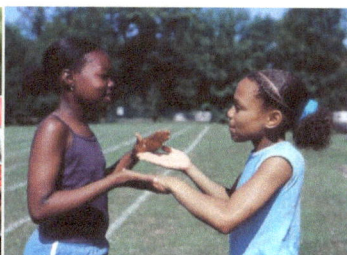

Billie Jean King

- Healthy younger adults about **7,000 to 13,**000 per day. (Lower for women than men.)

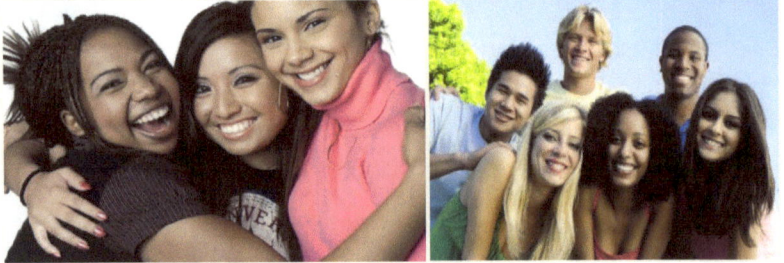

- Healthy older adults typically take **6,000 to 8,**000 steps per day.

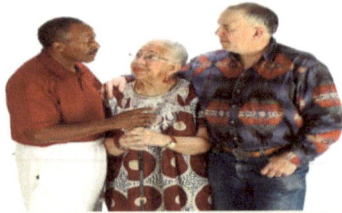

- Persons living with chronic illnesses or with disabilities typically take 3,**500 to 5,500** steps per day. The article concluded that the above steps need to increase to achieve optimal health.(To Read the entire article. Visit www.University of Arizona.com

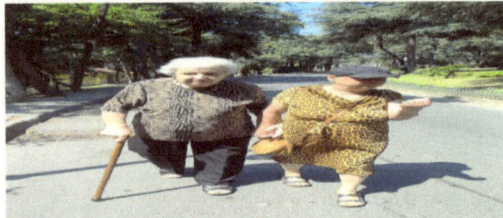

Environmental, Inherited or Social Contributors?

Although obesity is a common problem shared by most Americans; whether it's environmental, inherited or social, according to the Surgeon General, the problem is more prevalent and pervasive among Blacks and Hispanics. In the Surgeon General's Vision for a Healthy and Fit Nation, Jan. 2010, it was reported that: Among **40-50** year old women, about **52%** of non-Hispanic blacks and **47%** of Hispanics are obese; for non-Hispanic whites, the prevalence is **36%.** These differences also are seen among children and teenagers. For example, obesity is much more common among non-Hispanic Black teenagers (**29%**) than among Hispanic teenagers (**17.5%**) or non-Hispanic whites teenagers (**14.5%**).

Whose Responsibility Is It?

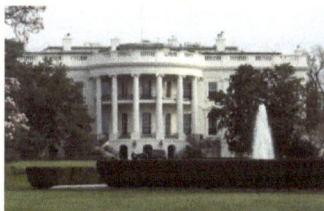 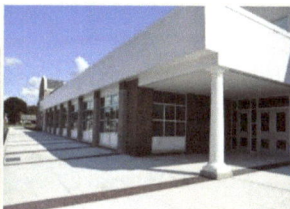 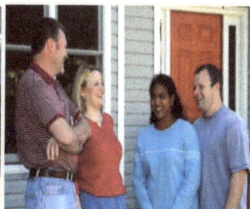

Government   Education   Parents

For years we've relied upon our educational system as being the accountability agent for enforcing the necessary physical activity for our children. I think we can all agree that the problem is bigger than our educational system can handle. Especially when some states and districts have limited mandates for P.E. programs at various schools. Consequently, it's definitely going to require a collaborative effort from health care organizations, food manufacturers, grocery chains, social groups, after school programs, and churches. As daunting a task that it is, unfortunately, the ultimate responsibility should begin at home with us as parents, grandparents, aunts and uncles.

Recently, this topic made its way to the political arena. Vigorous debates were raised concerning the topic of restricting the responsibility to parents only. I vehemently disagree. Individuals who feel passionate that it should be the sole responsibility of the parent are generally people with higher learning aptitudes, and are equipped with the knowledge and the finances that are essential in providing the proper dietary nutrients to their families. They fully comprehend the process in selecting the appropriate food groups that are conducive to planning and preparing healthy meals and snacks for their children.

In designated areas throughout the U.S., lunch programs for schools, daycare and after school programs will be the only place that some children will receive a wholesome meal. If the school system will lead the way for change by offering healthier choices in their breakfast and lunch programs; this would set a precedent to the parents by promoting an opportunity for them to incorporate the same recipes and entrees in their meal preparations at home.

Let's face it, if you didn't grow up in an environment that practiced and encouraged healthy food choices in meal preparations; the chances of you repeating the cycle with your kids increases. There are exceptions; some will break the mold as a result of higher learning, changing their environment, or by possessing a strong determination to make a change for themselves and their children, as with me. For now...there are more parents and households who need the assistance of our *government, schools, and churches to lead the way for them.*

As a nation, we've taken out too many things in the schools that were good for our kids. I clearly recall rushing to get in line for our school lunches. Looking back, our lunches were more consistent to a dinner. They were yummy, yet packed with nutritional value that would adequately grace the table of any Politian today.

Inspiration for Writing Book

"*This is going to be the first generation that's going to have a lower life expectancy than their parents,*" says Dr. Phillip Thomas, a British surgeon who works with obese patients. "*It's like the plaque is in town and no one is interested.*" *(American Chronicle, Paula Moore, July 9, 2007).*

Dr. Phillip's quote was echoed in an article stated by Shaquille O'Neal the following day. "*This is the first generation predicated to have a shorter lifespan than their parents. Childhood obesity numbers have tripled in the 20 years in the U.S. and nearly one-third of U.S. children; 25 million of them are overweight or nearly overweight.*" Shaq stated in an article by (*Willow Bay of the Huffington Post, July 10, 2007.*)

After watching Shaq's Big Challenge episode on childhood obesity that aired on **ABC in the summer of 2007**, I saw a little of myself in those kids. Struggling with my weight since childhood, the thought of my Granddaughter following in the same path sadden me. At the time, I'd been walking with a pedometer for three years. I recall one episode in particular; it was weigh-in-time. One of the boys weighed in and showed no weight loss.

Let's Get Steppin!

When questioned if he'd followed the prescribed activity instructions; he was unable to provide a plausible answer. I vividly recall playing the role of the coach sitting on the sideline, "*If they'd given them pedometers, they would be able to track their activity levels.*

This brings me to my story with Ashley, my Granddaughter, who was eight at the time. We began to notice that her weight was steadily increasing. Her Mom, like so many other Moms across the U.S. are genuinely concerned about the health and well being of their children. Always taking pride in preparing nutritional means; she decided to take it to another level. She began to spend more time in the grocery store aisles reading food labels; this prompted her to incorporate more whole grains, increased fruits, popcorn and less consumption of foods and beverages containing sugar, and high fructose corn syrup.

Since Ashley's Mom had grown up eating whole wheat bread; other whole wheat and grains foods came with little resistance. Ashley, being a pasta lover, and with extreme discriminating taste buds for an eight-year old; she was surprised to discover that whole wheat pasta was an acceptable alternative as well. A plan was in motion. Dining out was restricted; therefore, making mealtime preparations more of a priority than an option. Ashley loves salads and a variety of vegetables for a child. A second selection of veggies often replaced mashed potatoes or white rice.

From dinner invites at my place, she'd acquired a taste for brown rice, she had no choice. Her Mom also implemented portion control, an area by which I often received a slap on the wrist for allowing generous portions when visiting me. Bad habits are hard to break. You love to see kids eating their veggies and asking for more of everything.

Fast food...giving it up was [not] an option. This presented the biggest challenge. Since Ashley's dance class ended at 7:00 P.M. on Wednesday's, it was a designated fast food night, along with Friday, or Saturday. To avoid total deprivation and frustration, two nights of eating out remained on the table. After careful negotiations were completed, and I do mean careful, don't mess with the *fast food*. Sodas and shakes were no longer an option; water, and some juices were reduced to a small size or switched out for a salad or apple slices depending on the eatery. Between the two them, they'd struck a happy balance.

Since it was the winter season, her physical activity was limited to P.E. at school, after school daycare play and a once a week hour long rigorous dance class. In spite of the careful attention to meal time preparations, and alternate food choices, the weight was maintained, but showed no signs of weight loss. Nonetheless, their efforts for making food choices and changes were viewed as successful! After careful evaluations, it was concluded that increased physical activity was needed.

Pedometer Challenge to Granddaughter:

This is where I come in. Residing near them at the time; I got an *epiphany* to try the pedometer concept with Ashley. With Shaq's kids in mind, I thought, yeah, this would be a good time to try it on a kid. I figured that if it *motivated* me, then it would probably be a fun and innovative approach in creating more movement in her daily routine. Picking her up on alternate days when her Mom would work late; I implemented a work out regiment consisting of walking and jump rope. After purchasing her a pedometer, we took to the streets. Bursting with anxiety to try out her new gadget; she couldn't wait for me to drive to the destination to begin our walk. After exiting the car, she'd check her pedometer to make sure that it was securely attached.

At the time, what appeared to be every other step; she was checking her step count. With excitement and exhilaration, she would announce, "*I've walked X amount of steps.*" Since the pedometer wasn't worn to school, at the conclusion of our 40-50 minute walk; she would of course be shy of making her 12k goal, the daily recommended number of steps according to various healthcare advisors. Upon arriving to her home, and experiencing an adrenalin rush, she would ask, "*Can I jump rope; I have to get my 12k steps?*" Of course, this was music to my ears. Like me, she became so pumped and motivated that she desired to exceed her goal of 12k.

It's mid September, 2008, two months from Thanksgiving. In August, while purchasing clothes for back to school, she'd purchased a pair of cute blue straight leg jeans with cuffs that were too small. She was dying to fit into them; therefore, returning them was not an option. With about two and a half inches shy of fastening them; I seized the opportunity and presented her with a challenge toward fitting into them to wear on Thanksgiving Day with her new suede tan Eskimo style boots. With no hesitation or resistance, Ashley accepted the challenge.

In addition to walking and jump rope; she gave more suggestions for obtaining her step goal for increased activity and movements. Soccer-kick-ball, tennis, dancing, and boxing were incorporated into the routine as bonus steps. Sounds impressive? *Well...as not to discourage anyone, let me translate for you.* Our version of soccer was using a ball the size of a basketball. We'd drive to a neighborhood shopping plaza that had a huge parking lot. With safety in mind, and less traffic flow; we would park in the rear. This became her soccer field, a patch of grass or dirt enclosed by blocks of cement bricks became the goal post.

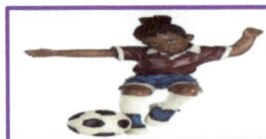

Let's Get Steppin!

*T*ennis: aw...my favorite, forever trying to live up to the name Billie Jean King, I always keep two tennis rackets and balls in the trunk of my car. This became her favorite activity as well. Armed with our pedometers; we'd take to the court. I knew that she wasn't capable of returning the ball over the net; but that was not my agenda. Increasing her step count on her pedometer was my goal. With each missed ball that I served to her; she had to run to retrieve it.

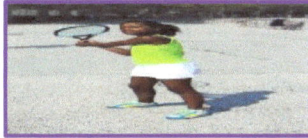

*S*he was so excited at the thought that she was actually playing tennis; she retrieved the balls with eager anticipation believing that she would return the next one. After serving balls over the net that were never returned; we would take to hitting the balls off of the wall, this was her favorite; and she was good. She would consistently return the ball from the bounce off the wall. After 40-50 minutes of ball running retrieval, Ashly would have racked up 5k to 6k steps on her pedometer. Feeling empowered and optimistic; she would beg to stay longer.

*J*ump Rope: another one of her favorites. My participation was limited only to counting her jumps. One hundred and fifty jumps were her goal. Challenging her that she couldn't do it twice; she accepted the dare and increased her step counts. She was eager to prove me wrong.

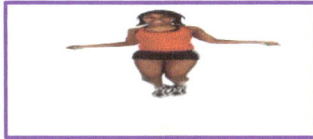

*B*y the end of October, after her weekly try-on session; her enthusiasm was off the charts. By sucking in her tummy; she was able to fasten her jeans. This provided her the hope and motivation needed in believing that by Thanksgiving Day, she would comfortable fit into her jeans.

*D*ancing: a favorite shared by us both. Residing in sunny California, in the winter months, it did rain on our parade occasionally. No worries, we'd take to the inside for some "private dancing." Private translates to not in public.

After setting up her Karaoke machine; we'd take center stage singing and dancing along with the medley of songs that came with her Karaoke. In her dance class, a new routine was always in the works. This became her time to show off her new steps from her dance class, and to incorporate some of her impressive choreography, which was actually very good. Please do not think that I was just standing idly by watching her, no, way, I had to show her that I still had some notable moves of my own, as we ramped up the steps on our pedometers.

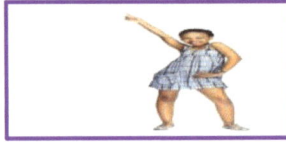

Boxing: her Wii video game proved to be another tool for activity and movement on extremely cold and rainy days. The game was rigorous and competitive. Employing a little Muhammad Ali demonstrated by me, her foot movement supplied her with the needed steps toward her 12k goal.

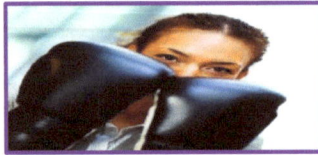

Basketball: Now, this was my favorite. It didn't afford me an opportunity for a game of twenty-one or anything close to it, but it did fulfill the purpose. Running down the ball after it hit the backboard did the trick.

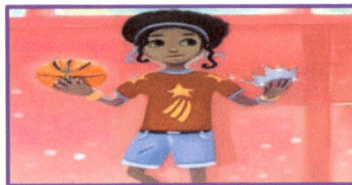

Let's Get Steppin!

I'm happy to announce that on Thanksgiving Day, she proudly wore her new blue jeans and boots to her aunts for dinner. The pedometer usage proved to be a positive method for increasing the movement and activity levels. The moral learned is, there are no boundaries when it come to creating movement and activity ideas.

Without using the work "diet," or weighing in on scales, we focused more on the number of steps taken in the course of the day. The food modifications and portions control that was implemented was a step in the right direction; weight management was controlled. Weight reduction did not occur until increased extra-curricular activities were incorporated into her daily routine.

In 2009, Ashley moved out of the area, which prevented the opportunity for us to continue our regiment. Ashley's Mom made a commitment to continue with the alternative food selections as a lifestyle for their household. Because of the lifestyle changes; Ashley's weight remains constant and is proportionate to her ever increasing height.

Since it's predicted that this generation of kids will have a shorter life span; will their nursing home expectancy age become consistent to that of their ancestors in the 50's?

While researching to speak to a group of seniors at a quarterly retirement luncheon; I came across this quote "*Today, the average age of someone moving into a nursing home is* **81.** *In the 1950's, it was* **65.***" The article was entitled, (***Is 60 the New 40 or 40 the New 60, by:*** *Lloyd Garver, May 2007.)* Since it's predicted that this generation of kids will have a shorter life span; will their nursing home expectancy age become consistent to that of their ancestors in the 50's?

3

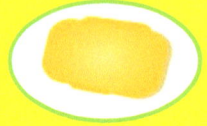

Notable Results: From Ashley Pedometer Challenge

After seven weeks of wearing the pedometer, the following was discovered:

- Her desire to engage in physical outdoor play increased immensely over watching the television.

- Attempting to reach her daily goal became additive.

- Wearing the pedometer was viewed more as a *game,* rather than a tracking tool for managing her movement levels.

Without resorting to food *deprivation,* and simply lowering her sugars, carbohydrate intake, and tracking the level of her activity proved to an effective method for weight management and weight loss.

Tracking her activity levels with the aid of the pedometer produced the following conclusions:

- Modified behavior

- Increased confidence and self-esteem

- Positive results inspired a desire for increased goal setting.

- Instilled a sense of personal accomplishment and fulfillment.

Let's Get Steppin!

Pedometer usage/Kids: Benefits to Parents:

Parents who are actively seeking ways to tackle and prevent obesity in their child, the following incentives and ideas [may] prove to be beneficial in making it happen for your kids.

- After reviewing the child's steps at the time of their arrival from school, or your arrival from work; depending on the number of steps your child have taken; you can immediately determine the type of meal to prepare relative to caloric consumption.

- If their activity level is sufficiently lacking, depending on the time of day, some catch up steps may be in order, e.g. treadmill, or their favorite walking or dancing DVD. To keep it fun and remain positive, give them the benefit of the doubt, just maybe, this was a no-fault day for them to reach their targeted number of steps.

- If the minimum steps and activity levels continue to be underachieved, depending on your child and your individual household rules, maybe a negotiable commodity can be introduced as an incentive for them to get their required steps before retiring for the evening. Choose something that will motivate them; a same day incentive award tends to be more effective, *promises...* do not work so well.

- Parents can make it a fun endeavor for the entire family. Friendly competition among family members to reach their goals can be an excellent dinner table discussion. *Friendly,* being the operative word; keep in mind that goals are individually based.

- After successful tracking, and activity levels have been achieved, yet, weight reduction has not occurred; this information can assist you in making the necessary changes in their food choices and portions.

- If all fails after food modifications, and movement levels have been attained, exploring medical complications with your physician maybe in order.

17

Billie Jean King

Summation of pedometer use with the kids:

The pedometer is currently being used primarily by dedicated adults who have taken a serious approach to achieve healthier bodies by tracking their daily routine. As we approach the next decade of the twenty-first century, hopefully the pedometer will mean to us what the *stop watch* meant to runners like Michael Johnson and Flo Jo, runners who raced against the *stop watch* to achieve their record setting goals.

Each of my pedometers were purchased from retail pharmacies. I think it's ironic that the pedometer is located in the wellness section along with the blood pressure and glucose testing monitors. Some retail stores will display them in their sports section. Still, several brands of pedometers are made by companies that manufacture wellness products. This should be indicative of the fact, that soon, the pedometer will be viewed as a medical device to monitor our health as well.

My purpose is to present an alternative support to parents and their children on the significance of placing more focus on increased physical activity within their daily practice; to make it a pleasurable approach to weight management and reduction while developing a life style of behavioral modification.

When we walk in our malls, amusement parks, work and school routes; we see cell phones, IPod's, or MP3 player's for every one out of three individuals that we meet. The day that we can visibly see a pedometer for at least one out of every ten individuals that we meet; we will then know that we've *"stepped"* in the right direction in conquering the war on Obesity.

The following charts will illustrate the activity levels tracked by kids in the course of their day, while at school, and playing their favorite sport. Based on the age of your child or children, I hope this data will assist you in gaining some perspective of the amount of activity that they are acquiring in a routine day.

Let's Get Steppin!

Recreational Sports Tracked by Pedometer

BOY- GIRL	AGE	ACTIVITY	DURATION	STEPS TAKEN
Boy	14	Football	45 Minutes	3500
Girl	12	Soccer	70 Minutes	3750
Boy	15	Basketball	20 Minutes	1500
Boy	18	Basketball	50 Minutes	4500
Girl	11	Tennis	60 Minutes	7500

STUDENTS TRACKED BY A PEDOMETER DURING AND AFTER SCHOOL

DAY	GIRL-BOY	GRADE	END OF SCHOOL STEPS	END OF DAY STEPS
Monday P.E.	Girl	4th	4500	6500
Tuesday P.E.	Boy	10th	14,478	14, 678
Wednesday No P.E.	Boy	10th	10,100	12,250
Thursday No P. E	Girl	5th	5800	7600
Friday	Girl	9th	12,450	13,558

4

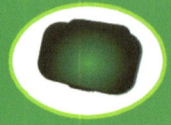

Wake up call:

While taking my morning walk; I received a phone call from my nephew informing me that his Mom, my older sister had been taken to the hospital via an ambulance after experiencing numbness. He was unable to provide me with a diagnosis until a series of tests were administered. It was later determined that she'd suffered a stroke, and lacked mobility on her entire left side. It's September 2009. She's insulin dependent with Type II Diabetes. Less than a year ago, in the beginning of the year she'd weathered a bout of pneumonia, and later was diagnosed with Sleep Apnea; joining my older brother who is also a diabetic with Sleep Apnea.

Taking queue from my nephew's calm demeanor; I felt that it was okay to continue with my walk. I must admit, the walking induced a tranquil and therapeutic state of mind at that moment. This brings me to my story of how tracking my steps with the use of the pedometer have impacted my life, and significantly reduced my risk for acquiring the diseases that are related to obesity. The call that morning was definitely a "wake up" call and confirmation that my walking was mandatory.

My Story: Pedometer Impact:

You know that adrenalin rush that you get when you find that half off sale, and you can't wait to tell someone about it, or discover that new product that's made a life altering change for you. That's how I feel toward this little gadget known as a *pedometer*. With my excitement level, you'd think that I invented it myself. Looking back, I can't recall who or how I was introduced to the pedometer. I just know that I began using it five years ago to monitor my walking. In the past ten years, I feel that I have a pretty good handle on choosing healthier food selections.

In 2005 I made a commitment to increase my walking regiment to seven days a week as opposed to three or four. Fitness Experts suggest that we should exercise at least three to four days a week. I figured that if four days a week is an acceptable amount to support good health, well, six to seven days should give me some *bonus points*. Both of my parents died of congestive heart failure, and I must add that they both were far too young.

Let's Get Steppin!

My Dad passed away at the age of 64, and my Mom at age 72. Unfortunately, their heart disease stemmed from unhealthy eating which lead to Obesity. I'm a firm believer that obesity takes on the form of being a *"generational curse,"* a curse of **bad eating habits** that can be broken. Now you see why I need to walk seven days, those extra days are not *bonus* points, they are sustaining grace points. I'll elaborate later on in the chapter.

My Pedometer Journey:

After researching usage, and the functions of the pedometer; it was suggested that to secure a five mile a day walk, **10k** steps were needed. *"Ten thousands steps, five miles, that's a lot of walking, I grumbled."* I had increased my walking time to an hour, so I was curious to determine what my step count for an hour long walk would be. The first day I averaged 7k steps, the second day, and 7.5k. I began alternating between 7 to 7.5k steps daily. It didn't take me long to figure out that the count varied depending on my stride and pace. If you're an avid walker, you're probably saying, *"is that all she walked in an hour?"* You guessed it, I'm a slow walker. I place more emphasis on endurance, rather than speed. It will be different for each individual.

Walking with or without a buddy:

If you're just beginning to walk and contemplating the idea of getting a walking buddy, you may want to give the idea some serious consideration. If you're like me, and have extremely short legs; it can pose a problem for your walking buddy if they have the capability to take longer strides. More than likely it would be a friend or family member, which mean that they would be kind and try to hold back their stride to accommodate you. If they are a serious walker, it could ultimately become frustrating for them. In my attempt to keep up with my walking buddy, I also found it difficult to carry on a conversation. I needed the extra oxygen to maintain my pace. For this reason, I enjoy walking alone, plus it's an excellent opportunity for me to reflect on the issues of life. If you're successful in getting a walking buddy, and both of you wear pedometers; do not allow the difference in your step count to discourage you. Keep in mind, if you began your walk together and finished it together, no matter what your pedometers register, *you can have the confidence in knowing that you both walked the same distance.*

Like a little kid with a toy I found myself taking frequent glances at the pedometer. I had mapped out a distance that would generate me 8k steps or more. After about two weeks of usage I was able to pinpoint my 2k and 3k step points along the route, and taking fewer peeks at the pedometer. In times past I viewed walking as a prescribed recommendation from my doctor. Now, it's like I'm on a mission, I feel as though I'm walking against time.

Billie Jean King

In the midst of walking, I enjoy my reflecting while focusing on the surrounding beauty of the trees, grass, and flowers. It's inspirational, encouraging and motivating to see other walkers as well; it's also affirmation that you're doing the right thing. Without striking up a conversation with each and everyone that you meet, yet, there's a sense of unity and agreement that's exchanged when you're greeted with a nod, a smile, or a robust good morning.

Dividends in sight:

Following a month of committed walking for six to seven days a week; I noticed a difference in my breathing. I wasn't as winded when my walk ended. To avoid discouragement, I opted not to weigh myself while using the pedometer. I decided to let my clothes be my witness. Boy, did I have a testimony. My clothes were getting a little baggy, while some were less tight, depending on the size of them.

Depending on my appointment schedule for the ensuing day, oftentimes my work involved me driving to an appointment and then sitting. Consequently, I generally ended up with a deficient of 4k steps needed before retiring for the evening. Getting a brainstorm, I remembered a walking DVD that was given to me by my daughter a few years back. The maximum walk time was three miles, displaying each mile completed on the TV screen. Watching a group of women and one man step in place for 30 to 40 minutes became boring. Since the man was in the infant stages of his weight reduction, even he wasn't an incentive to watch. I'm sure his purpose was to be an encouragement for other men, and not to entice the viewing audience of women such as myself. To keep me motivated, I would listen and step the music from my MP3 player.

By the end of the day, I had reached my 12k to 13k steps on most days. Listening to my MP3 player while walking keeps my focus off the length of time that I've walked and more on ramping up my walking speed. The pedometer definitely gives me the incentive and drive needed to make it through my morning walks. By watching the steps increase on my monitor; I'm less compelled to keep watching my watch. Looking at my pedometer excites me, the numbers on it move at a faster speed than the minutes on my watch, so, I no longer wear one.

On the days that I would leave home without my pedometer, and was too far to return to get it; I would literally become frantic, concerned that I would lose account of my activity for that day. To ease my frustration, I had to remind myself that if I walked the exact same course, with a steady swift pace that I would still accomplish my required steps. At the end of the day I only needed to add the estimated morning steps to the remainder of my steps.

Let's Get Steppin!

After five years of committed walking at 6:00 a.m., this year I took it to a higher level during the rainy season, and boy did we have an extended wet season. As a consciousness walker, the first thing that you do is peek from the window to get a visual of the day. In past times when it rained, I would I take the attitude, I'll just walk tomorrow. But this winter rain continued into the early spring in California, it appeared that no tomorrow was in sight for walking. It didn't rain the entire day, but, some days included a constant drizzle. After going two days without walking, I began to get nervous, and you know what follows nervous behavior, yeah, eating.

While peering from the window, I noticed that some of the people that I would meet on my route were walking with their umbrellas and rain gear. New to the neighborhood, I thought, *"Hmm, now these are some serious walkers."* You guessed it, I'm now rumbling through closets looking for my hiking boots and umbrella. You know…, it wasn't so bad; I'm not talking thunder storm rain, but the kind that was depicted in the famous Gene Kelly scene. Yep! I danced and sang, just for a second; I couldn't resist.

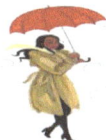

I have to confess, the six to seven days of walking has resulted more on the weight maintenance side than weight reduction. Earlier, I mentioned the "bonus points" for walking seven days a week as opposed to three or four. Well, when I've consumed an excess amount of calories, the extended days are no longer considered a bonus, it becomes a balancing act. And that's not a bad thing depending on your agenda.

As I previously pointed out, I'd gotten a handle on making healthy food choices. Converting to whole grain breads, pasta, and brown rice, I exclude white foods as bread, rice, potatoes and pasta. I also avoid processed meats, cold cuts, frozen cooked foods and foods high in cholesterol. Deep fried foods such as chicken and fish are restricted to social events for my eating pleasure. When cooking at home my meats are stir fried, grilled or baked. I eliminate breads that include *enriched flour (white flour)* and food and drinks that are made with tran's fat, hydrogenated vegetable oil, and high fructose corn syrup. To cut down on sodium consumption, I substitute salt with herbs, spices and other salt substitutes that's on the market. Although salt is a necessary nutrient, it's also a harmful one if you're trying keep your blood pressure lowered. Eating out has been the biggest challenge, especially with American based restaurants. Vietnamese and Indian restaurants offer you a choice of white or brown rice.

When choosing the brown rice, when I make wise meat and vegetables selections; it becomes guilt free eating. I attribute these types of changes to the success of my weight management. You'd be amazed at how good the whole gain foods taste. In addition, you're guaranteed a *natural elimination* within 24 hours. Sorry! Per Dr. Oz, *if we maintain a steady diet including whole grains and fiber, we should be eliminating the previous 24 hour meal daily.*

Aw...sweets, they're my weakness. What is known as a yogurt parfait has become my choice of dessert. Except for those days that I go to the market and can't pass up that individual slice of German chocolate, or carrot cake that's on sale for $1.99. And what's a slice of cake without some ice cream...yum. Thank God for our good friends *Ben & Jerry, Hagen Doz and Dove,* they were thinking of sweet lovers like us when they introduced their line of the 2oz. cup serving of ice cream to satisfy that nagging craving. You may be thinking...ooh she's bad. No! *Bad was when I used to buy the half gallon of ice cream, and the whole cake, and consume it all in 3 days.*

"Good" Can Be a Hindrance:

You're familiar the expression, "too much of a good thing can be bad for you," or something like that. Most of you will probably agree with me that I made some serious food changes as well as behavior modification. So, the question becomes, in addition to all that walking, and good food choices, why wasn't I losing the weight. It's all about the big "P," Portions. I'd been consuming food in portion sizes that were not conducive to weight loss. Because of the walking; I've been able to maintain.

Being a bread lover, at times, I would trick myself into baking loaves of whole wheat bread. This was to insure that I would be getting 100% whole wheat bread with no possibility of it including any enriched flour, nice theory, but it was also certain that I'd eat the entire loaf within two days. Because the foods were whole grains, and not "simple carbs," they didn't convert to sugar and fat after consumption; instead, combined with my daily walking regiment, it provided a balance and prevented me from gaining weight.

Walking with an Agenda in sight:

For my class reunion in August, 2009, I went on a "reducing diet" to lose weight to coincide with my daily walking and step monitoring. The operative word is reducing. I can't resist defending the poor little four letter word, **diet.** For so long we've used the word diet out of its proper context, until, now, we're being instructed by some not to use it all together. It's almost considered a bad word these days.

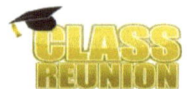

24

Let's Get Steppin!

How often do we say, "I'm going on a diet?" Whether we choose to use it correctly, or not, the meaning of the word diet will always exist as being the sum total of what we eat on a daily basis.

With my class reunion in sight, I carefully implemented portion control, and ramped up my walking pace and time. I increased my daily step goal to 13-14k, depending on my schedule. I was successful in my attempt. Well, enough in the sense that I was recognizable to my classmates and family members. Since then, my weight remained constant, it only fluctuated two or three pounds over a period eight months.

How Quickly We Forget:

It's been about eight months since my sister's stroke. With no agenda in sight; I'm coasting along and keeping my weight steady. Ordinarily, that would be considered a good thing if I had already attained the recommended weight needed for [my] body frame. But, since I'm forty to fifty pounds overweight, I can't afford the luxury to just maintain any longer.

I'd forgotten the wake-up call from my sister's stroke, which is still in the restorative and rehabilitation process. I'd forgotten my eighty-four year old aunt whom I care for weekly that takes eight to ten pills daily attempting to manage complications from the related diseases stemming from obesity. I'd forgotten about my other three siblings, uncles, aunts, and a host of cousins that's suffering with type II diabetics, heart disease and hypertension. My six month check-up had produced me a clean bill of health; I think I allowed it to give me a false sense of comfort in thinking that by comparison that I was doing alright, Not! In spite of my juggling act with whole grains and consistent walking; my present weight still keeps me in the high risk category to contract diabetes and other diseases.

I have not made a full scale commitment to consistent portion control, and to avoid certain sweets that continue to enslave me. In my fifties, I know that it's only a matter of time before I will no longer be able to engage in an hour long walk, or jump around my living room dancing to the beat of music from my MP3 player, which aids in keeping my sugar, blood pressure and cholesterol levels low. I realize that I'm only prolonging the inevitable. Still relatively new to my neighborhood; I was still experimenting with various walking routes. A month ago I'd lost my pedometer, without the use of the pedometer I couldn't pinpoint my step count. Losing it is a topic that will be discussed later.

Surprisingly, I didn't panic, I knew I had another one; it was only a matter of me locating it. I later discovered that it was in a box that was still in storage. Since I'd considered upgrading my pedometer anyway, it was much easier to purchase another. This meant going online and checking my options. When I completed my search, I decided to purchase it from a major local retail pharmacy. I kept it simple, limiting it to two functions. It monitored steps and a five day memory capacity in case I forget to write my steps on a given day.

To my surprise, the route that I'd been walking for a month without my pedometer *only generated me about six thousand steps*. Now, panic sets in. I couldn't be assured that my activity level was conducive to supporting my balancing act. To obtain some sense of affirmation and assurance; I pulled out my monitor and checked my blood pressure levels. It registered 130 over 80. Not bad, I reminded myself that I'd probably induced it a few numbers by my present state of anxiety. After re-taking it thirty minutes later, it registered 125 over 75; this for sure was more comforting.

With the aid of the pedometer I was able to immediately isolate my problem area and make the needed adjustments in my walking and daily activity; as my blood pressure monitor provided me with assurance that my pressure levels were okay, my pedometer made me aware of how off track I'd become by not monitoring my daily movements.

I can't give enough praise to this little *gadget*. I'm amazed at the assurance and confidence that I get when I'm wearing it. When I'm consistently tracking my steps, I do not feel the need to constantly weigh myself. I have the confidence in knowing that if I hit my daily goals, I'm stepping in the right direction. I'm gradually climbing my way back to 12k steps a day. I've refrained from baking whole wheat bread or evening buying a loaf. Certain temptations *I have to avoid entirely*. Until they decide to sell bread by the slice; I settle for a few whole grain crackers to satisfy that carb craving.

After carefully planning my daily diet, implementing portion control and increased walking; my body is now in the mode for my weight to reduce. Easier said than done, with no special incentive or event in sight; it's become a real challenge. You know how we are, when we have that special occasion coming up and vanity creeps in, making it easier to meet that weight goal. *I had to finally face reality; my incentive needed to be focused on staying healthy for **life**, and not only during specified periods of life.*

Can Sacrifice and Denial Be a Good Thing?

I guess you can tell by now that I [love] good food. The mere thought that one day I may be [denied] the opportunity to enjoy it with all the savory seasonings that make it taste so good; hmm…I shudder to think. A dear friend of mine shares my sentiments.

We've decided that if we want to continue to enjoy good eating at every stage of our life; then there's going to have to be some sacrifices along the way. If you dance to the music, you got to pay to the piper. Simply put, exercise!

This is a perfect example of sacrifice and denial. Mild cheddar cheese is one of my favorite snacks. I love it with crackers, bread, grapes, or just slicing it and eating it. I love the thick 8oz pack. I could eat it every day, but I know that I can't. For the past ten years or longer, I buy it *once a month*. When I first started, I found myself writing the date down in anticipation of eating some more. And yes, I would eat it all the same day. After waiting for a whole month; I felt a sense of entitlement. In the last few years I haven't had the urgency to purchase it every month. When I do buy it, I know that it's okay, because oftentimes it's been two months since I've purchased it. I think setting the once a month guideline took away the feeling of deprivation. You may think, wow, that's extreme, maybe, but it worked for me.

My total cholesterol levels have remained between 128 and 140 for the past fifteen years. I'm reminded of a previous co-worker who'd gone to the doctor and became ecstatic when she discovered that her total cholesterol level was 275. We began to share our numbers, at that particular time mine was 128. She shouted, *"no way!"* but her tone and expression said, *but you're bigger than me.* She looked to be a slender sized 8. She and her boyfriend dined out frequently, she'd always bring leftover lobster drenched with drawn butter and a steak. Is this scenario comparable to the age old controversy of, *can a person be overweight and yet, healthy*? Can a thin person with high cholesterol levels of 275 be classed as healthy?

Facing Reality-Choices:

The reality is, for the remainder of our life, we will always be faced with the temptation to eat sumptuous foods. The decision is; how will we deal with it? *Unless we've been instructed or advised by our physician to abstain from certain categories of food; we do have some choices and options.* The following illustration will speak volume.

27

Billie Jean King

Facing Reality-Choices, continued:
I think our health care professionals are saying:

"If we dance to the music... from over indulgences...

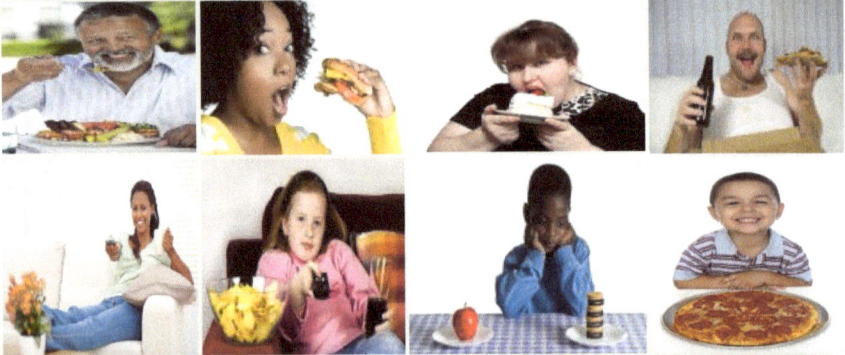

We've got to pay to the Piper ...Movement & Exercise"

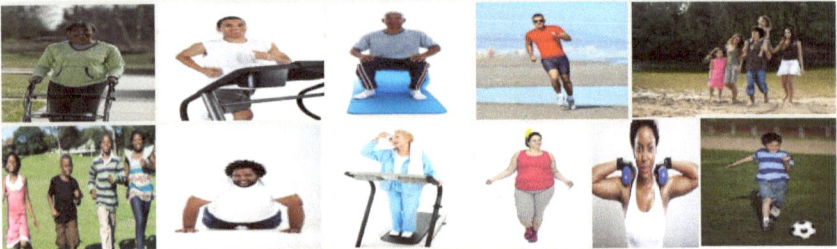

Or ...Come Visit US

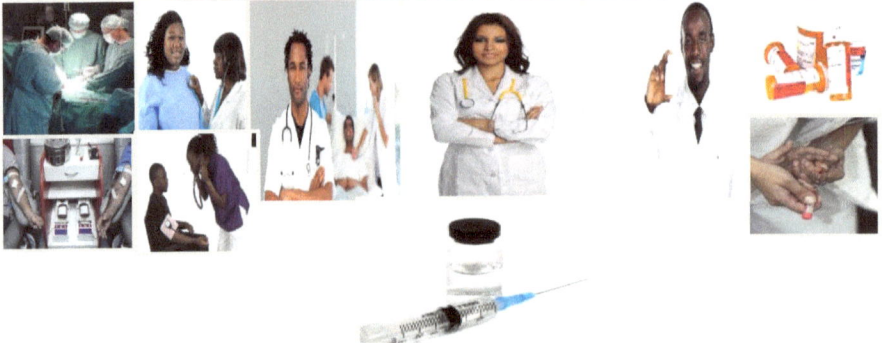

28

Let's Get Steppin!

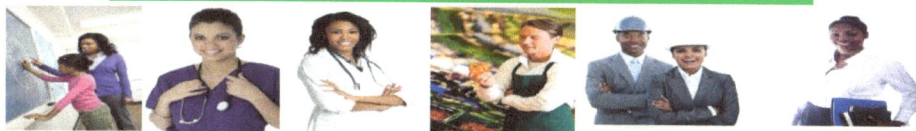

OCCUPATION	GENDER	DURATION	STEPS TAKEN
Window Clerk	Female	9 hr.	7500
Retail Store Manger	Male	10 hr	9100
Electrical Engineer	Male	8 hr.	9500
Mechanic	Male	8 hr.	4500
Admin Asst	Female	8 hr	4950
Medical Doctor	Male	9 hr	8500
Dentist	Male	9 hr	6500
Bank Teller	Female	8 hr	5501
Recruiter	Female	8 hr	4350
Director of Social Ser-vices	Man	8 hr	4150
Nurse	Female	8 hr	9500
Grocery Clerk	Male	8 hr	5800
Bank Security Guard	Female	8 hr	6500
Insurance Agent	Female	8 hr	5500
Teacher	Male	8 hr	5890

29

Billie Jean King

100 ADULTS SURVEYED
ON PEDOMETER AWARENESS – USAGE

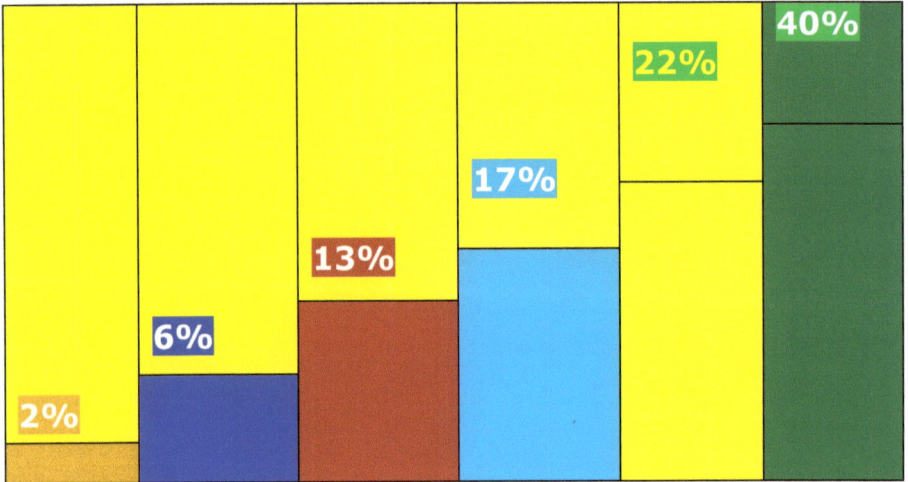

2%	Never Heard of A Pedometer
6%	Received Free-Used for Short Period
13%	Received Free- Never Used
17%	Purchased- Use Occasionally
22%	Purchased-Use Daily
40%	Received Free – Use Frequently

30

5

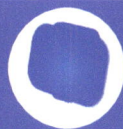

Leading by Example:

Not only should we as parents and grandparents encumber the responsibility to lead by example for our children with good nutritional habits; we should also feel a sense of obligation to bear the burden in providing encouragement and assistance to our siblings and family members as well. Just as there's always a "black sheep" in the family, it's generally a leader also. You know that relative that is respected as being wise, a counselor, mentor and or advisor.

My aim is to step into a leadership role in reaching out to share with my family the simple changes, and adjustments that are sustaining me with a reasonable portion of health. It will also keep the spotlight on me and challenge me to propel to the next level. I've appointed myself to be an advocate to help my family. If I win the lottery, or the PCH prize; I wouldn't hesitate to share my winnings with them, I feel the same with matters concerning our health.

Whether you've heard a convincing testimonial regarding a particular product, or seen live footage from an infomercial product, or maybe you're heard a heartfelt testimony from a member of your congregation; they're all designed as encouragement to get you to take action, which is my agenda.

Intervention to family:

My first goal or phase is to get my family moving; implementing food changes will be the second phase. I'm providing them with pedometers to give them a clear snapshot of their movement levels. I'm not limiting it to my siblings only. Since a kid, for four generations I've witnessed the same health issues, therefore, I'm extending it to my family members in the south as well.

I've teased and joked with my family in Louisiana regarding the ensuing story. When visiting last summer for three days to attend my class reunion; my family took me to a local Chinese Buffet for a Sunday Dinner. I will repeat, a Chinese Restaurant. Thinking to myself, "W*ow, they've become citified, just like Californians.*" This is my home town in *Louisiana, home of southern* and *Cajun* style cooking. I'm visiting from out of state, after 20 years "*and they take me to a Chinese Buffet… for [Sunday] Dinner, that's blasphemy.*"

31

Before arriving there, I can assure you that I'd entertained many thoughts of me *wrapping my lips* around a *Sunday Southern* style dinner. I knew the "*throw down cooks*" in that of my older aunts were no longer with us; but...I had hoped that some of my cousins would carry on the tradition. Not!

In a minute you'll see the significance of the buffet dinner story and why I felt compelled to include them in my "Let's get Steppin" Campaign. A few months ago a series aired entitled "*The Food Revolution*," hosted by Jamie Oliver. In one particular episode, Jamie visited a school cafeteria. On this particular day he pointed out the fact that everything on the menu was *golden* in color. This included fried chicken nuggets, chicken strips, tator tots, and French fries. The camera scanned the food displaying steam tables loaded with *golden brown* food. Instantly, I had a *flashback*.

When dinning with my family members at the Chinese Buffet; one of my uncle's daughters', who sat across from me, made an observation and decided to voice it. Referring to my plate, she stated, "*Wow, she's the only one that's eating healthy with vegetables on her plate.*" This prompted me and my cousin seated next to me to quickly scan the long table that we were seated. She was correct, as far as our eyes could see; every plate was filled with *golden brown* food.

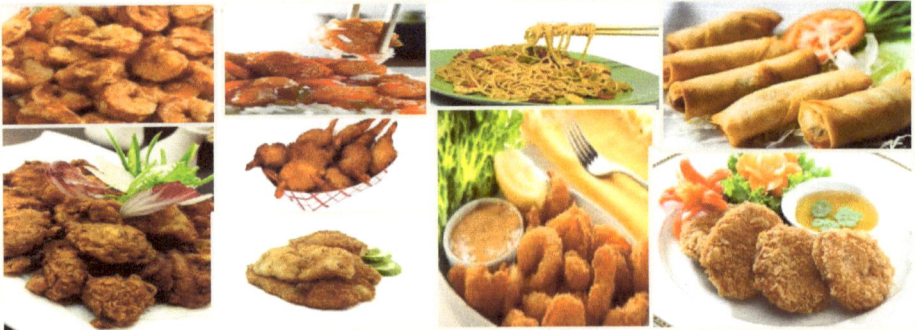

Her statement was acknowledged in agreement and swiftly dismissed with a hearty round of shared laughter. I hope you picked up on my cousin's expression that she used when she referenced the vegetables, "*eating healthy.*" More than often we know what foods that we should be eating. Rather than balance our food choices; we tend to gravitate toward those foods that taste best. In their *defense;* my plate included *golden food* as well. I must confess; the food was *yummy*!

Let's Get Steppin!

F ull *redemption* was in order when one of my cousins later informed me that he was off work the Friday that I arrived. He assured me that if he'd known of my arrival time; he would've prepared me a home cooked meal complete with his well known BBQ. Hmm…guess who'll be picking me up from the airport on my next visit?

Holidays Dinners-Menu Changes:

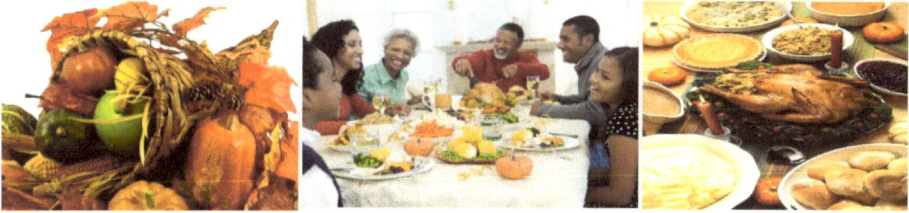

S ince the early seventies, Thanksgiving Day Dinner, Holiday BBQ's were a given to be hosted by my sister and her husband. For Christmas, we do our own thing. In light of her stroke two months prior; she was out of rehab and on her road to recovery. I think everyone in our family would agree that 2009 Thanksgiving Dinner invoked a deeper sense of thankfulness. Gratefulness that wasn't limited to her just being alive, but that her mobility level allowed her the *privilege* to be able to sit at the dinner table and engage in conversation and laugher as in past years.

Talking about a reason for gratitude, I'm sure she'd be the first to express appreciation for finding a husband who is a great cook also. In the past three to four years, her two young adult son's interest in cooking was peaked after watching TV personality Chef, G. Garving. Timing is everything, between her sons and husband; we didn't miss a beat that Thanksgiving. Understandably, with respect to my sisters' condition, there was a need to incorporate necessary menu changes. Fortunately, we were able to continue with the traditional spread of foods. After receiving the invite that the dinner would take place; my first thought went to food considerations for her. Being on a no salt diet; I knew this meant extra time and preparedness. Not to worry, the boys came through.

Since the turkey and stuffing was the desired entrée, a separate pan of stuffing was made with herbs and no salt seasonings. A high grade turkey roasted in its natural juices and a few spices provided a satisfying taste without salt.

Billie Jean King

Along with a toss green salad, collard greens and baked yams for her dessert, she was able to enjoy a satisfying meal without feeling deprived. Without sacrificial preparations and selfless menu changes on her husband and son's part; she would've been *tempted* to eat foods that were restricted from her diet.

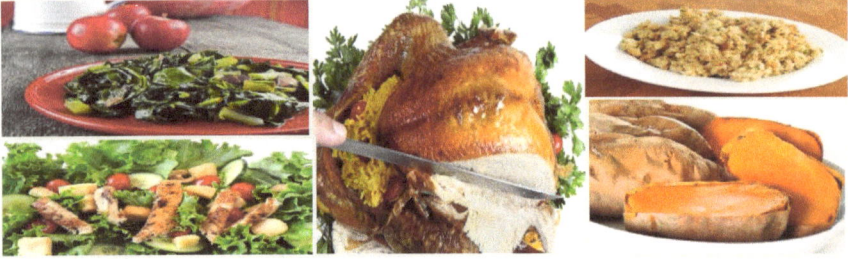

At dinner time, using a **teaspoon,** I dished up a spoonful of stuffing, collard greens and a piece of turkey. Loving bread, I grabbed two small squares of cornbread. Within five minutes, I was at the dessert table cutting my chunk of cake and slice of pie. My daughter baked a four layer coconut cream cheese pineapple cake. I baked my favorite sweet potato pie. Remember choices, if you dance to the music, you pay to the piper. I'm Miss Sweet tooth, so I knew that I wanted a big of chunk that cake and a generous slice of the sweet potato pie; the choice was easy.

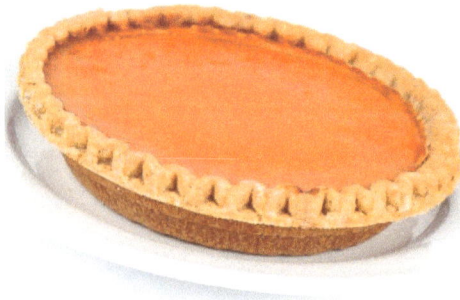

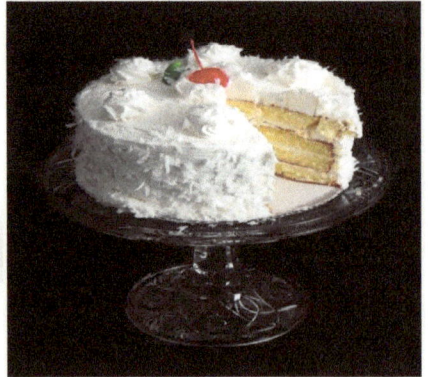

I'm happy to report that I only had a second slice of pie. *These are the type of extreme sacrifices and denials that I've come accustomed to employing when I have to choose yummy desserts over everyday regular food that I can get anytime.*

Let's Get Steppin!

Family BBQ's- Change in Venue and Menu Considerations

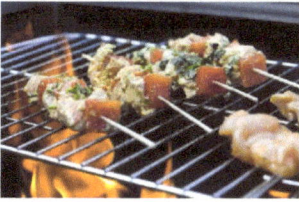

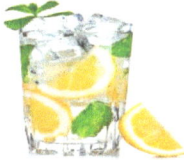

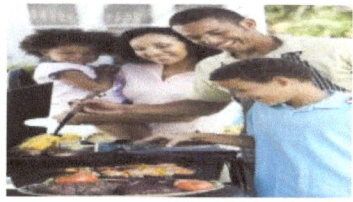

Traditionally, Memorial Day is the first BBQ holiday to kick off the summer season, hosted by my sister's husband. After getting up at five o'clock in the morning to fire up the grill, by ten o'clock a.m., the meats would be grilled to perfection and simmering in steamers for added tenderness.

When we didn't get an invite for Memorial Day, in 2010, we knew it was time to pass the torch of holiday dinners and BBQ's to the younger generation. Caring for my sister, cooking, and related chores were shared by both nephews and my brother- in law; however, the day to day tasks did not offer them the luxury to prepare for continued holiday entertainment. Did I mention the fact that he's 86, and still going strong. I guess his secret is having a wife twenty three years his junior.

With over thirty years of family gatherings in their home, my daughter and I knew it was time for a change in venue. In past times, my daughter and I would complain about the fact that our family in California is so small when we'd hear of other families and their big gathering. But, when it comes to food preparations, small is a good thing.

Earlier in the year, my daughter had purchased another home; without question, she knew that she was next in line to be the designated host for our holiday events. The next holiday was the 4th of July. You know how we do it, ribs, chicken, hamburgers, hot dogs, beans, salads, corn on the cob, desserts. Consideration for my sister went to the top of the menu planning. To be fair to everyone and to avoid denial to her as well as the other guests; she a planned menu tailored to my sister's food restrictions. In light of the fact that my daughter is an excellent baker, everyone including me wanted one of her delicious cakes. She settled on a three tier yellow and chocolate cake.

What's cake without ice cream, remember? In past years, my sister would make homemade ice cream for the summer holidays. Yep! That was added to the menu as well. We knew that she couldn't eat the cake or the ice cream, and a yogurt parfait would've been considered cruel by comparison. In the final analysis, my sister's menu consisted of smoked chicken and beef ribs seasoned with herbs and tons of no salt spices, a tossed green salad garnished with jumbo prawns, and corn on the cob.

For dessert, my daughter prepared a special batch of homemade vanilla ice cream made with *Splenda and 2% milk.*

Words alone cannot adequately capture the sense of satisfaction, thankfulness, and appreciation that resonated from my sister's countenance. She was amazed at how pleasing the meats were to her pallet. The ice cream, she was past ecstatic, it was a real treat. She suffers from sweet tooth weakness too.

It was a good day. Our biggest fear was that we would experience guilt while she felt deprivation. With a little consideration, organizational skills and multi tasking; we pulled it off. When preparing her meats we immediately identified it with colored tooth picks. Believe me, they were a life saver after all the meats were placed on the grill.

For future family gatherings; we realized that consideration, time and preparation will be essential in providing a proper balance for everyone. As for me, I headed straight for the cake and ice cream. While helping with the grilling; I'd tested a bite of most of the meats, so when it came time to eat, my appetite wasn't craving meat. Plus, I knew that the meat would be around the next day, the cake and ice cream, not!

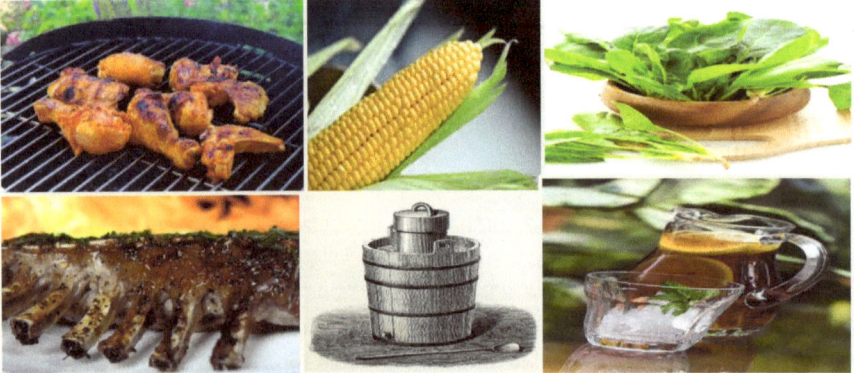

6

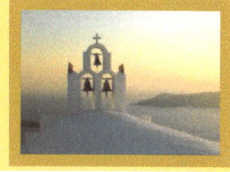

The Church-It's Impact on Obesity

The church today still remains the cornerstone by which we as Christians cling to for spiritual guidance, comfort and support. Whether it's a mega church with a congregation of thirty thousand, or the neighborhood store front; they've all opened their doors to feed the needy during this recession. More progressive churches have offered financial relief as well as housing for some of their members. Unfortunately, the needy are no longer limited to the homeless. Parishioners are finding themselves on the receiving end of a ministry of which they once were a financial contributor. No matter the level of support, *it's a reassuring thought to see that the churches are practicing what they teach and preach.*

Stemming from the end of the 20th Century; the church was no longer viewed as an institution for worship only. As a new generation of Pastors emerged, they adhered to the mandate and took to the streets in their communities to grow their congregations. The fruits of their labor were rewarded by a harvest of new converts. This became a two-fold blessing; some Pastors were able to walk away from their nine to five job.

This growth wasn't limited to the Pastors position only. By the early eighties, it was common on a week day to drive by a local church and find the parking lot occupied with cars other than the Pastor's preparing for his Sunday sermon. Depending on the size of the congregation, you'd find a full time Assistant Pastor, Janitor, three to four Administrative Assistants, a full time Youth Pastor/Director, and a Director of the Outreach Ministry/Evangelism. The church had come full circle as an establishment that created employment opportunities consistent to small business owners.

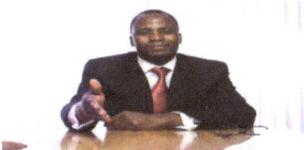

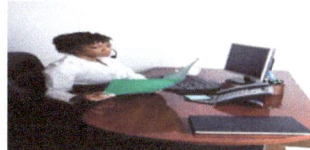

Today, some churches can be compared to corporations with the Pastor being the CEO. This level of abundance had long been shared by various nationalities, *but, within the ethnic communities, it definitely was and is a new day.*

Billie Jean King

As growth in attendance increased; the traditional Sunday School Book was supplemented by teaching materials that focused more on spiritual growth. Titles such as auxiliaries were replaced with more *purposed* minded titles now known as the singles ministry, men's ministry, women's ministry, youth ministry, young adult, senior's ministry , and so on. Each shares the same purpose; to be nurtured, and to grow in the admonition of the word. Lastly, but certainly not the least, to have fellowship (food), one with another. When more ministries were introduced, the more opportunities became available to *eat and fellowship.* As congregations grew, it also generated revenue abundance, which in turn, afforded more food to be available for fellowship gatherings.

To share a little history, as a kid growing up in the south during the sixties, church fellowships were always celebrated with a spread of holiday style menus. Very few churches were equipped with kitchens, so, our parents tried to bring their kitchens to the church. They would literally bring large boxes that would hold containers of fried chicken, potato salad, stuffing, cakes, pies and all the trimmings. I know you're thinking, "*how did you heat it up?'* You didn't, if you were lucky to get in a line with someone that was a *great cook;* as long as it was good, you'd be so hungry by the time you were served; you didn't care about the temperature of the food. Unlike now, kids eat first. Uh, kids got in line behind the Preachers and anyone that looked like a preacher in my day. This background information was shared to highlight the history of the church and its association with food and the financial progression of the church, and how it has *unconsciously* aided in the advancement of obesity.

Today, we're equipped with not only industrial sized kitchens; some have fully operational cafeterias. Additionally, others have dining areas that include large flat screen televisions. As churches continued to thrive and progress; it ushered in more opportunities to fund fellowship events. When finances were not available, various departments coordinated potlucks. Not all, but some churches prepare breakfast between Sunday school and the eleven o'clock morning service. Again, not all, but some are serving up fried chicken, fries, potatoes, biscuits, waffles and the works.

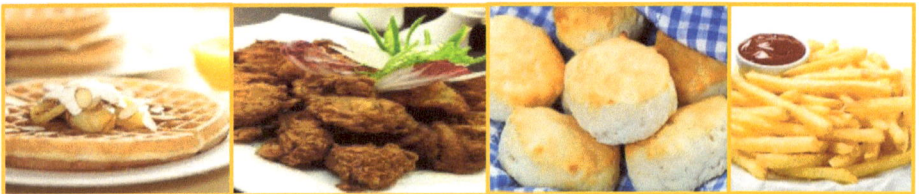

Random Survey to Churches:

placed a random call to a group of churches across the U.S., in appreciation of them sharing, I will employ anonymity. When asked if they served breakfast and if so, what did they serve; the menus varied. Continental menus consisting of yogurt, cereal, bagels and cream cheese, do nuts, pastries, orange juice, and milk was a favorite. Others were more consistent to the above menu, including sausages, eggs, pancakes, oatmeal, grits, fried chicken, bacon, and ham. When asked about their evening youth fellowship events; pizza, soda, buttered popcorn were the overwhelming favorite, with hot dogs coming in second.

With adult fellowships in mind, spaghetti & meat sauce, lasagna, fried chicken, tossed salads, bread sticks, cakes and pies were the top entrée's for evening events. Favorite potlucks entrees were spaghetti and meat sauce, beef taco salads, meatballs, mac & cheese, collards greens, and meatloaf.

Churches with large screen televisions and fellowship halls come together to watch sports, or provide movie night for the kids. The menu can range anywhere from pizza, buttered popcorn, hot dogs, fried wing dings, French fries, BBQ, cookies, sundaes, sodas and hot chocolate. Since we have four major sports in that of basketball, football, baseball and hockey throughout the year, it's feasible to see how the pounds could began to mount. When it comes to churches; I think that we can mutually agree that fellowship appears to be *synonymous with food.*

In 2010 Dr. Ian Smith intervened [at the request] from some parishioners of a church that was preparing a weekly Sunday breakfast consistent to the food selections in my survey. It gained national attention on the Oprah show. He passionately challenged and informed them of the serious health consequences from their indulgences. I found it odd that there were no men featured during the entire segment. I know that the ratio for women to men is disproportionately high within the church, but no men... which bring me to my next topic.

It's estimated that about 60% of church attendance is held by women. The make-up includes widows, divorced, married, singles and singles with children. Studies suggest that unmarried women of faith tend to embrace food for emotional comfort in the absence of a male relationship. As a single woman...Hmm, I will stipulate that it has some merit, but we're not alone. Wives tend to gravitate toward food as a comfort method to cope when there are troubled waters in their marriages. Unless men are just plain old greedy; *they are not excluded from emotional eating.*

Billie Jean King

Gluttony: The Forgiven Deadly Sin:

Since the church is the authority figure for promoting obedience to the scriptures; I feel that my appeal is in order. With that said, it behooves the church to step up its effort in preparing sermons that highlight and identify "Gluttony" as a sin that destroys the body [*temple*] to the point of death. Since eating is a daily requirement for sustaining life; Gluttony tends to get a *pass* in relation to other overt *sins*. Think about it, we will openly identify *adultery* as being the consequence of sin in a failed marriage, or a *pregnancy from fornicating*, or death by a *drug overdose*. Have you ever heard anyone say that an obese person died of a heart attack, diabetes, kidney failure, or a stroke that was induced by the sin of "Gluttony?" Never..It's become the acceptable *silent, but deadly sin.*

Since fellowship among like minded believers play an integral role in the life of a Christian, while serving as a social mechanism it's also an essential means to keeping one encouraged in their faith. Therefore, the need for Pastors and leaders to perform series evaluations concerning their contribution to the health and well being of their parishioners should be of paramount concern.

Teaching and preaching about gluttony from the pulpit is definitely needed, but it must be followed up with application and example by providing healthier food alternatives. *Let's face it, obesity is not a problem for everyone, and they should not be denied the enjoyment of culture culinary delights of which we've grown accustomed.* However, options for healthier choices should be made available for preventative measures against obesity and those members with known health conditions. You may argue, *the church can't decide for them when they go to their perspective homes.* This is true, *but the church in a good conscious state can't be guilty of creating an environment and the opportunity for the very thing that they preach and teach against, [temptation].*

Once food options have been made available to escape the *temptation*, then the decision rests solely on each individual. Hopefully, a nudge from a concerned sister or brother will suffice when they speak, *"C'mon now, you know you don't need that, how about this choice instead.* To validate the previous paragraph; I'm a witness that when alternative food options were made available, it opened a door to escape the *temptation* without feeling deprived or denied. Bear in mind, as stated in my introduction, I remain in this struggle with you. Therefore, I'm not preaching, but crying out for help on our behalf.

40

Let's Get Steppin!

To get your congregation moving this summer; on a voluntary basis, consider organizing a pedometer challenge for the summer months for all age categories of your congregation. Set a goal for the number of steps you'd like for your church to go on record achieving. The target amount will be based on the ages and the number of participants.

- To keep everyone engaged, retrieve weekly step counts. Reports can be retrieved via the Sunday school hour, children's church, women, and or men ministries, etc.

- For vacationers, or apprehensive starters, allow anyone to join at anytime.

- To prevent discouragement from over achievers and competitiveness; do not record steps using individual names, but, by age group or category instead.

- Design a huge board visible to everyone to see the challenge when entering the sanctuary.

- Designate a coordinator for each group to submit the weekly totals to be entered onto the Master Chart.

- Set your target step goal for the summer months based on the participants and recommended steps for each age category.

Utilize the expertise of your healthcare professionals within your church, *remember always check with your doctor before beginning any exercise regime.* To assist you in gathering your data for your chart, (refer to chapter 2, steps taken by age groups.)

SUMMER PEDOMETER STEP CHALLENGE SAMPLE CHART

Wk	AGE 6-12	AGE 13-18	AGE 19-30	AGE 31-40	AGE 41-50	AGE 51-UP	Totals
1		300,000	450,000	440,000	420,000	385,000	285,000	2,280,000
2								

JUNE'S STEP TOTAL: _?_   SUMMER TARGET: _?_

Billie Jean King

What Some Churches Are Doing To Combat Obesity:

I saved the best for last. From word of mouth, and a few surveys, some churches have taken a serious approach to providing a holistic type of ministry for their parishioners. The following are examples of what some churches are doing to incorporate healthy eating habits while helping to combat obesity; beginning with annual health fairs that include diagnostic screening of blood sugar levels, blood pressure, cholesterol, and weight.

- Vendors that specialize in alternative food and beverage products.

- Pamphlets and brochures stressing the importance of walking and daily exercise.

- Several churches are offering morning and noon day walking teams.

- Others provide free after work onsite workouts and complimentary health bars and bottled water.

- Classes are offered teaching the importance of label reading to ensure that you're selecting the proper foods.

- For children events, bottled water is substituted for sodas. Subway sandwiches cut in ¼ portions along with turkey burgers are provided over hot dogs when affordable.

- Menus for luncheons are being exchanged with salads garnished with strips of chicken, or turkey served with a roll, bottle water and an energy bar for dessert.

- Women's, and singles ministries breakfast functions are serving oatmeal, yogurt, bagels, bananas, cereal, turkey sausages, fresh fruit and bottled water.

CHURCH HEALTH FAIR:

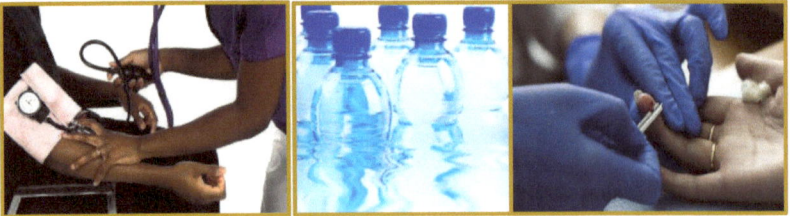

Church Community Gardens

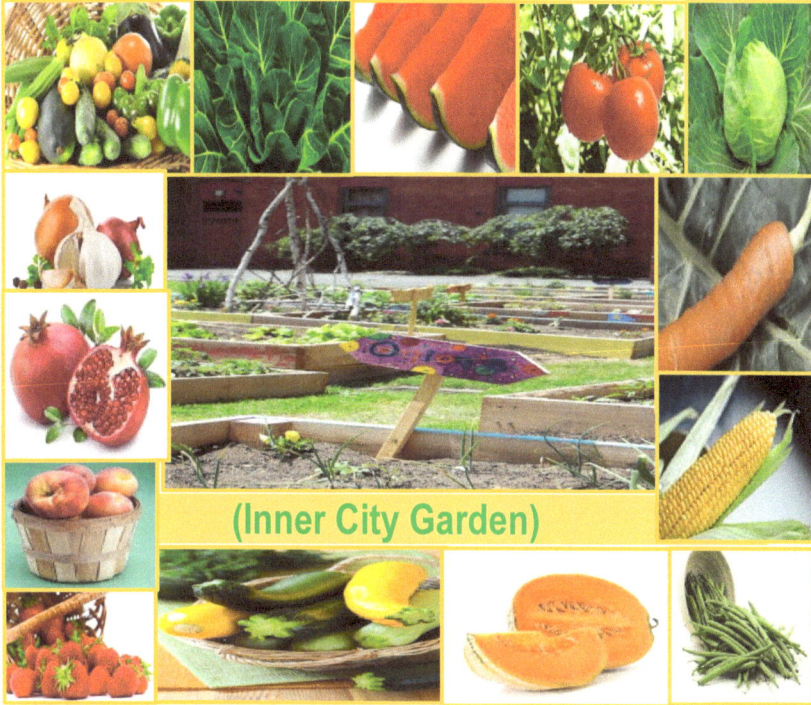

(Inner City Garden)

This time last year homes and community gardens were popping up everywhere after First Lady Michelle Obama sphere headed her garden at the White House. And what a great idea it was. In my unsuccessful attempt; I tried planting some tomatoes, reaping a harvest of only five delicious tomatoes.

It's a known fact that the inner city communities are under serviced when it come to supplying the residents with fresh produce in the grocery stores. It's also appears to be a matter that can't be regulated by government officials. If families are denied fresh produce by the markets that serve them; *why can't churches lead the way in helping to solve that problem as well?*

There are two establishments that remain constant on the corner or in the middle of the block in every urban or inner city neighborhood, a *liquor store and a church*. It may not be enough land on the church property to plant a garden, but surely there has to be a member that own a home with a backyard; or maybe there' an empty house with a backyard that can be rented by the church for the purpose of gardening.

43

Surely Churches that are attempting to feed their parishioners and neighboring families must be feeling the pinch when it come to purchasing fresh vegetables to serve with their meals. With a little bit of planning and coordinating, churches can host a community garden for their parishioners and neighborhood residents. Since most churches are equipped with Vans for picking up kids and the elderly for Sunday morning worship services; the same concept can be orchestrated in picking up kids and individuals to work in the garden. In the eighties, community gardens in urban cities of Chicago were a huge success, as the one illustrated previously.

Can you imagine the pride and a sense of accomplishment that would be realized after seeing a harvest of fresh grown produce? Not to mention the tasty and healthy meals that could be prepared. Many churches hand out weekly bags of day old bread and pastries that's donated from local supermarkets. Wouldn't it be great if the church could hand out a bag of *free* fresh grown vegetables along with the bread and pastries?

Until we can dig our way out of this recession; *I'm convinced that the Church will play an even greater role in the sustainment of families across the U.S.* Unfortunately, certain entitlements that should be afforded to every community in America is beyond the scope of demand for elected officials. Fortunately, with a little ingenuity and elbow grease, supplying families with fresh produce from church hosted gardens is something that's within the compass of being achieved.

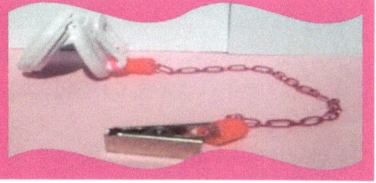

Secure your pedometer/with a safety leash

Last, but certainly not the least. In light of the benefits and usefulness of the pedometer; it does need assistance in remaining secured to your waist. This is the only down side, it will drop from your waist. On most occasions you will hear it fall to the ground; but, if you're walking on grass or on a soft surface you may be unaware that it has fallen off. Ladies, girls, if you're wearing pants, the most common place to drop it is in the bathroom, after you unfasten your belt… men too. Any bending or twisting motion can reposition the grip to your garment, causing it to drop later.

Fashion Pedometer Leashes:

In the past five years I've lost two pedometers. Forever possessing an inquisitive mind; I began to explore the possibility of creating something that would secure the pedometer to the garment. Like most ideas, you ponder them for a while before they end up in your mental file, labeled "*later*."

One day while ordering some pedometers from Amazon.Com to give to individuals for testing; a safety leash for the pedometer popped up as being an item commonly sold to pedometer customers. Of course I didn't purchase it at the time, but I did take the time to contemplate the idea and studied it with intense curiosity.

After careful examination of the safety leash, I knew that I could improve upon the one that was being offered. Improvement as it relates to aesthetic, appealing to the eye, and a more user friendly clip for arthritic users, the elderly and smaller kids. It received great reviews from customers validating the fact that a safety mechanism of some sort was definitely needed. Since kids were my initial inspiration and focus in promoting pedometer usage; I figured a more colorful and fashionable device would be more suitable and appealing to them, especially to girls.

In consideration to boys and adults; I chose less dazzling shades of black and silver. After researching to see what pedometer colors that were available on the market; I was delighted to find that they come in colors of red, green, pink, yellow, purple, blue, orange and black, consistent to cell phones and IPods cases.

As I pondered the idea, I began to see visions of colorful chains corresponding to the identical colors of the pedometers that I had earlier discovered on Amazon. The baffling part is that; I had *not seen any color chains in the market place.* There were lanyards, ropes, and cords in every color of the rainbow. My pursuit for colored chains in the dimensions that I was seeking was limited to stainless steel, and gold. I could not shake the image of the colorful chains from my brain; so the search was on. I'm happy to share, after many Google searches; I found my color chains, and my *patent is pending.*

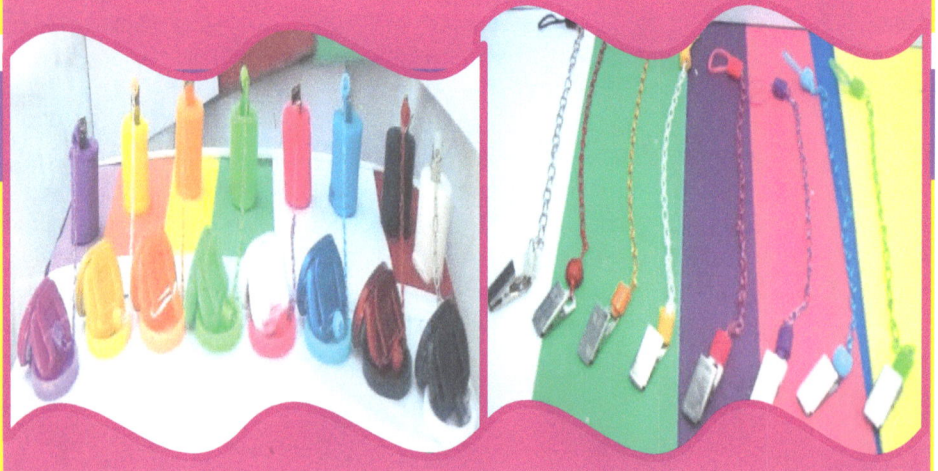

8

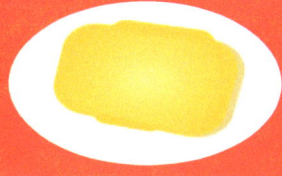

Effects of Simple Carbohydrates-Fats-Sodium-Cholesterol

It is said that education promotes empowerment and open doors of opportunity for change to occur in the life of an individual. I'm a firm believer that when conscious minded people become informed and educated on the role, cause and effect that various foods and additives play in determining the quality of their health and mortality; change will be welcomed.

I will refer to this chapter as my extreme overview. Seeing is believing, it is said that a picture is worth a *thousand words*. I'm reminded of a friend in the 1980's who subscribed to Ebony Magazine. While visiting her home one day, I saw an article on the front cover that I wanted to read. I said, *"I need to subscribe to this."* She replied. *"Don't bother, you can have mine, I never read them anyway. I only like looking at the pictures of the hairstyles and fashions. It gives me ideas and keeps me up to date."* Although she didn't read the articles, yet, the visual illustrations were powerful enough to resonate in her memory and for her to achieve her purpose.

When your eyes set sight on the following food illustrations; I hope the visual effects will serve as a subliminal reminder when you walk the aisles of your favorite grocery store. It's my intense attempt to show you the devastating effects of various food entrees; such as processed and manufactured foods that we ingest daily without awareness. The following images will depict the foods that appear on the breakfast, lunch and dinner tables of families of all nationalities and social-economic status across the U.S. Some of us eat these foods without a conscious thought of how they are impacting our health and well being.

Did you know that white flour based foods become sugar, and later act as stored fat once they enters into our digestive system and blood stream?

WHITE
FLOUR   *SUGAR*

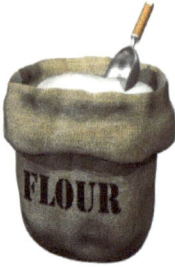

FAT

=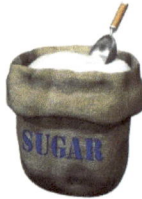

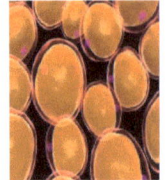

Did you know that your favorite can or bottle of soda contains

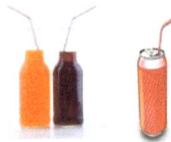

12 to 14 teaspoons of sugar?

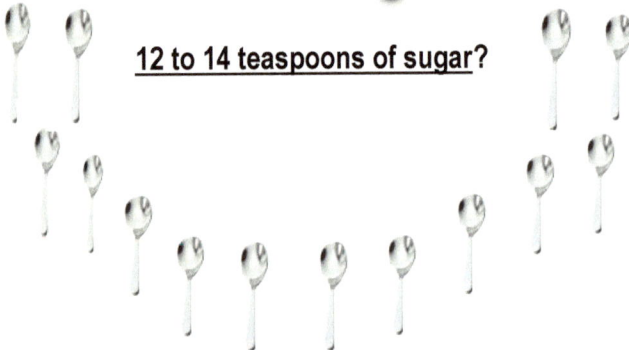

White Flour Based Foods- Simple Carbohydrate
(Also High in Fat and Cholesterol)

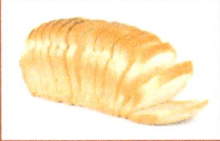

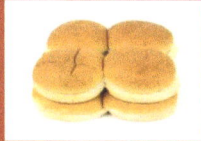

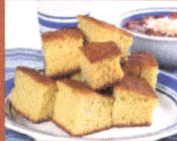

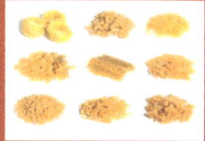

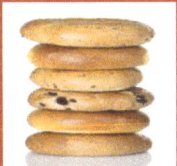

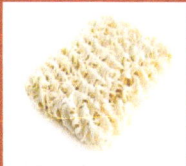

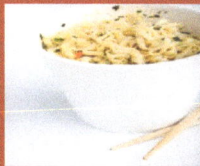

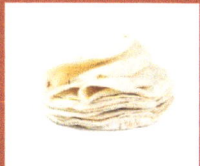

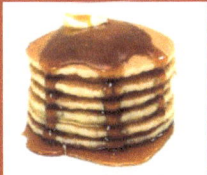

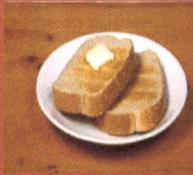

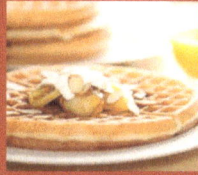

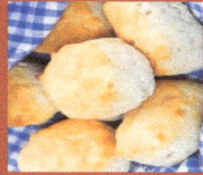

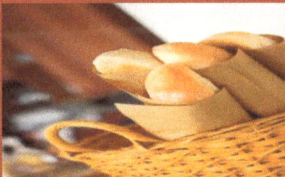

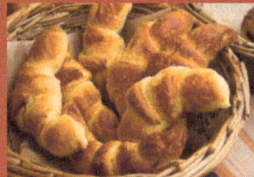

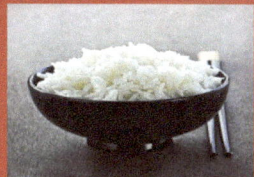

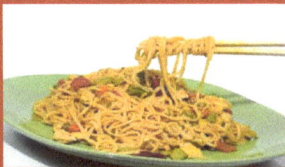

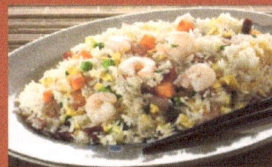

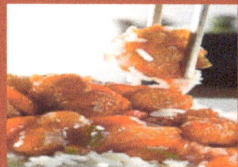

Flour Based Foods-Simple Carbohydrates Continued:

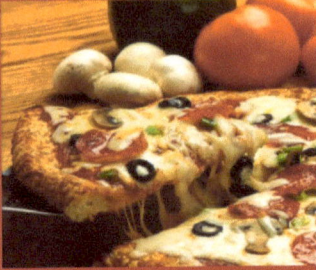

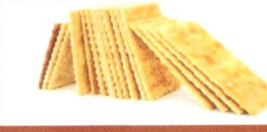

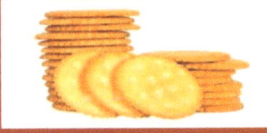

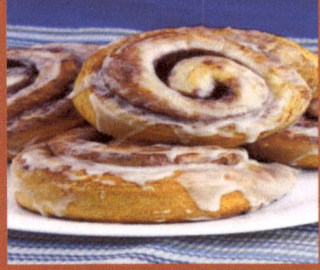

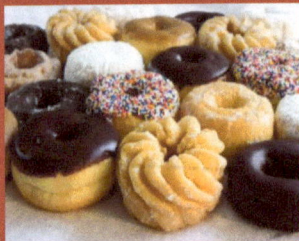

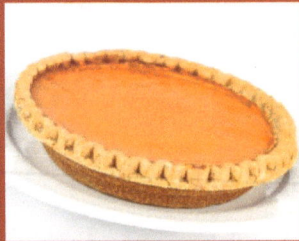

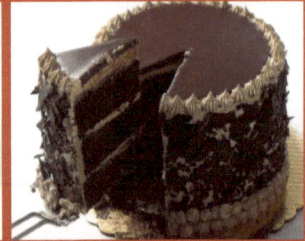

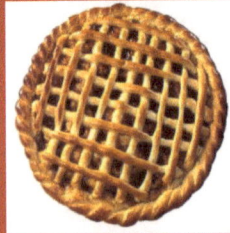

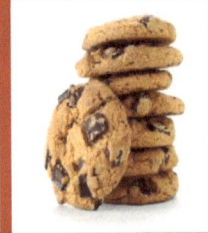

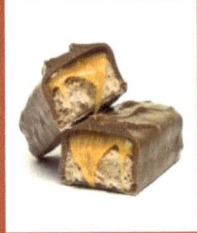

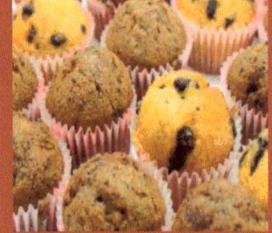

Billie Jean King

Foods High In Fat- Sodium-Cholesterol

Fried Chicken

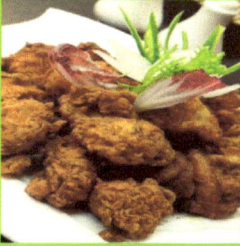

Chicken Nuggets

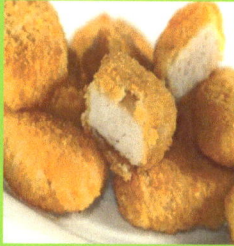

Cream   Cheese Bagel

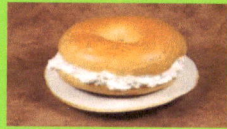

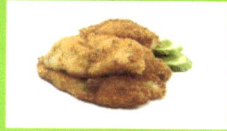

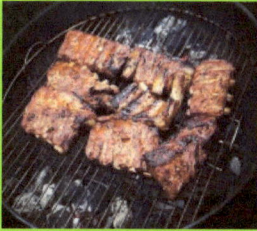

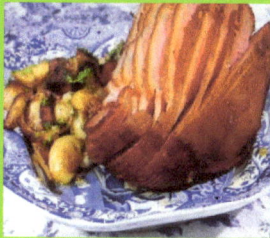

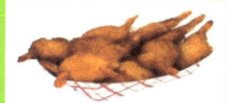

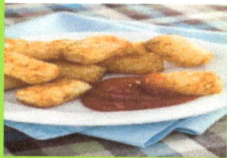

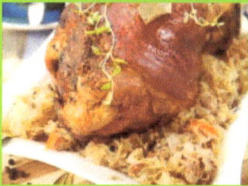

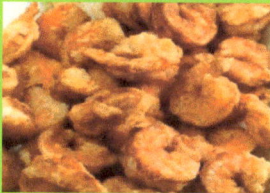

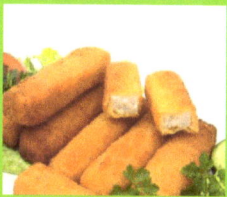

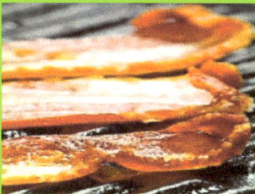

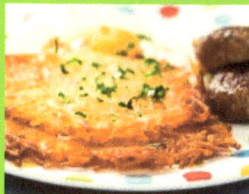

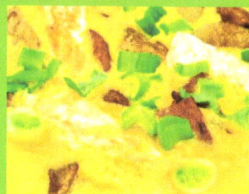

Bacon

Hash Browns

Omelet

56

Let's Get Steppin!

Foods High In Fat- Sodium-Cholesterol

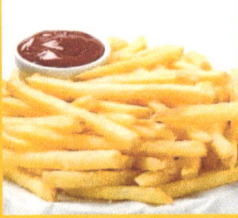

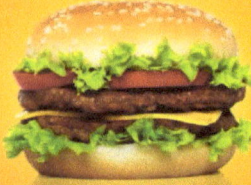

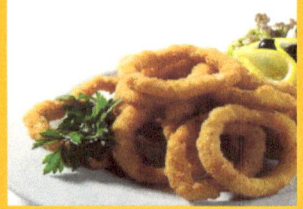

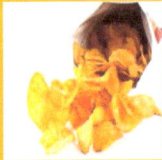

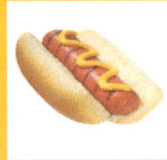

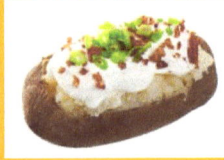

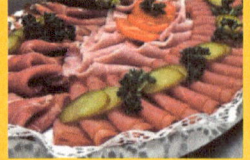

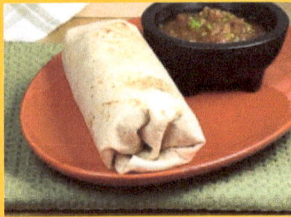

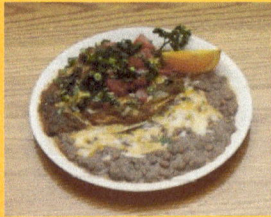

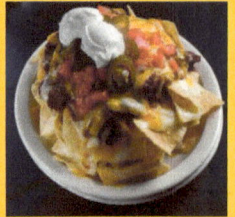

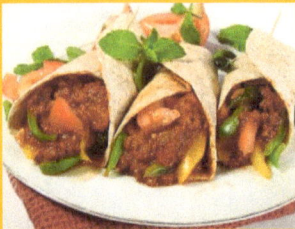

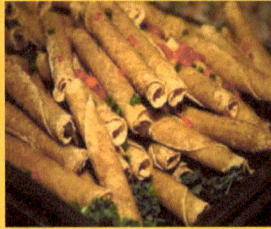

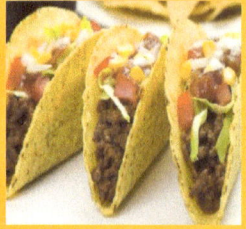

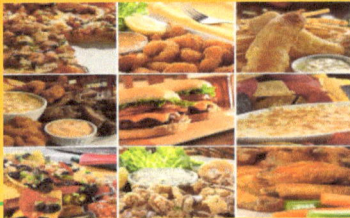

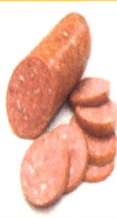

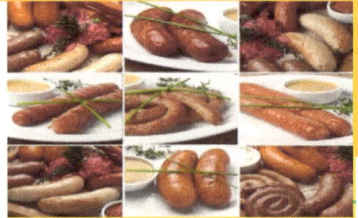

57

Foods High In Cholesterol-Fat

Whole Milk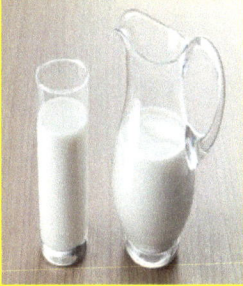

Mayo

Salad Dressing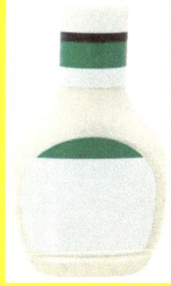

Butter Milk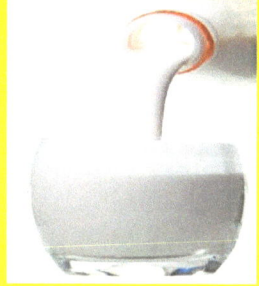

Potato Salad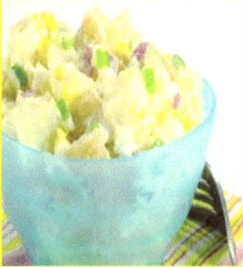

Lasagna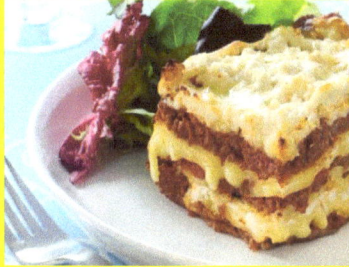

Mac & Cheese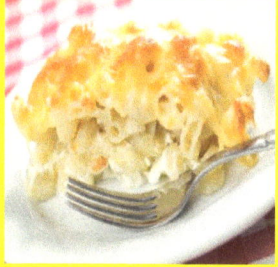

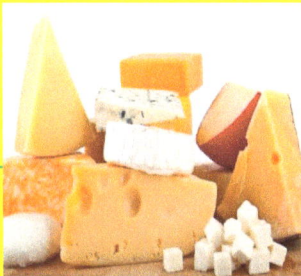

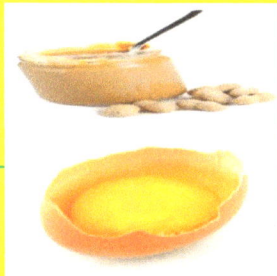

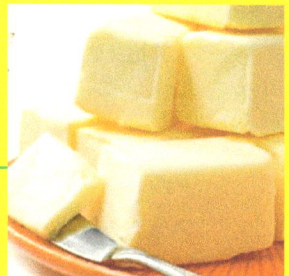

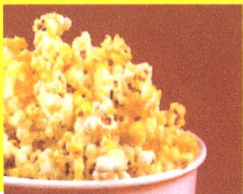

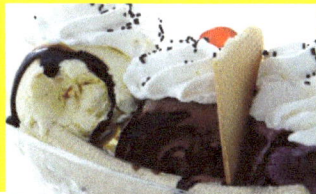

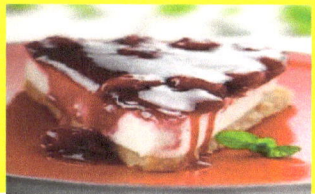

Let's Get Steppin!

According to an article published by helpwithcooking.com "simple carbohydrates consist of one or two sugar molecules, which means that due to their simple structure, they can quickly and easily be broken down into glucose and converted into energy very soon after they have been consumed." It further state that "sucrose is the sugar we use to sweeten our hot beverages and it is also present in cakes, pastries, soft drinks and sweets. It is also found in other processed foods, which we may not be aware of. This type of sugar, the unnatural kinds, is what makes us put on weight, not to mention causes tooth decay, mood swings, hunger, lack of concentration, **diabetes and hyperactivity, especially in children.**"[Excerpt taken from: helpwithcooking.com, Copyright 2001-]

Per Dr. Oz, in and of itself, sugar does not make people fat. Cells in your body burn sugar from starches, fruits, and sugar as fuel. Excess sugar is stored for future energy needs in the form of fat.

Further clarification on sugar and simple carb's effects stated by Dr. Doris Day; The more simple sugars you eat, such as in candy, the faster the sugar ends up in your bloodstream and the more insulin gets released to control it. First, the sugar is converted to glucose. What happens next is that the increased levels of insulin by the body as it tries to regulate the blood sugar level leads to increase production of fat which is pushed into the cells as storage for later use. Glucose is the main fuel of the body. We convert fats and carbohydrates to glucose as we need it in order to have the energy we need to live. However if you eat too much of simple sugars and other simple carbohydrates, or foods with a high glycemic index, you increase your risk of weight gain, lower your energy levels, and run the risk of type 2 diabetes and other health problems.

Why We Need To Read Labels:

[Unsalted] Tops Cracker

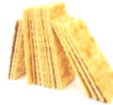

Did you always think that unsalted meant that the crackers contained NO SALT? Well, I did too. After a discussion concerning food labels and their ingredients with a friend; she challenged me to read the label on a box of *unsalted tops*. I was shocked and mortified after learning that SALT is one of the main ingredients. I always wondered why they tasted so good.

UNSALTED TOPS refers to the fact that there is no salt on the TOP of the crackers, as with the saltines. *SNEAKY!* Since salt is included in the ingredients; why is excess salt needed on top of a cracker anyway? The operative word is TOPS.

Before my Mom crossed over she was on a sodium free diet, unsalted tops were a part of her weekly diet. This was twenty years ago; we trusted the outside wording. This is a perfect example of why we need to read labels and why manufacturers need to be held accountable for their role in confusing consumers. If you're supposed to be on a NO SALT diet and you are eating "unsalted tops" regularly, it will explain why you're having problems getting your blood pressure lowered.

9

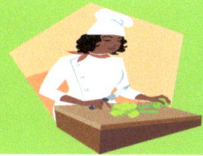

Alternative foods and recipes for healthier eating:

By now, I know you're saying, "*is there any food that's good for us.*" As I stated previously; too much of a good thing can prove to be bad as well. As Americans, we've come to love everything SUPER SIZED, including our portions at meal time. Therefore, some of us have exhausted our privilege to choose wisely, instead, we have to abstain altogether. In this chapter, I've complied some of the foods and recipe alternatives that I attribute with keeping me *diabetes free* thus far. My primary struggle now is **portion control.**

When it comes to changing eating habits or trying new foods; most of our apprehension stem from the dread of how it will taste. *We do not like change.* When my granddaughter was in preschool, at mealtime, a strict policy was in place. Before the student could refuse to eat a particular food, they had to have a **"no thank you bite."** What better age to teach open-mindedness. I thought, what a brilliant idea and a lesson that we all could benefit. Think about it, our taste for the foods that we eat and love are cultivated from an environment of what's prepared in the home, extended family members homes and friends. Consequently, we learn at an early age to avoid foods that look different from that which we are accustomed.

At the age of about six or so, I was a guest for dinner in the home of a non-family member. Banana pudding was served for dessert. When asked if I wanted any, since it wasn't a familiar food to me; I recall staring at the dish of pudding. My Mom to that date had never prepared a banana pudding for us. I loved bananas, but the cookies and pudding over showered the bananas. Reluctantly…I tried it, *and it was the best tasting stuff that I'd ever eaten at that age. And, today, remains one of my favorite desserts.*

Since adapting to whole grains and brown rice; honestly, the taste of white sliced bread and white rice is extremely difficult for me to swallow, literally. On occasion I will ask an individual "*do you like brown rice?*" Often time their response is "*yuk! Or no!*" I then ask "*have you tried it?*" More than often the answer is "*no, it's not what I'm used to eating.*" Before saying no to new food choices, remember the "*no thank you bite;*" it just maybe that food that will promote good health and longevity of life.

Let's Get Steppin!

I will start with breakfast. That's supposed to be the most important meal of the day. Let's be real, when it comes to traditional foods that are eaten at breakfast time, such as bacon, sausages, ham, and omelets, that are filled with the same meats and cheeses. Then we have stacks of pancakes, French toast and waffles, all made from white flour; this can't be considered a healthy prescription to get us going in the mornings.

Have you noticed how breakfast is the least expensive food on the menu in restaurants, and... it's the meal that restaurants routinely offer ongoing specials. Generally the specials consist of pancakes, eggs and pork meats of your choosing. You can find these specials everyday in every city. Yes... they're priced with *recession consciousness*, but frequent consumption of these foods will return dividends that will result in poor health. It's the convenience that's get us. *We all know that if we can afford to eat out... for just half the cost, a more nutritious breakfast could be prepared at home;* even if it only consisted of cereal and milk, or a hot bowl of oatmeal.

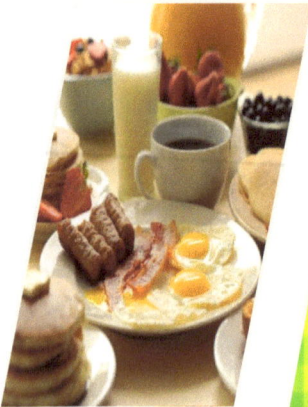

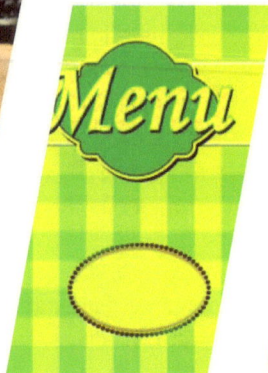

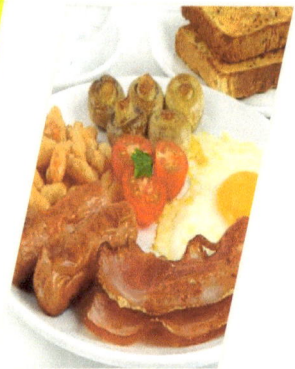

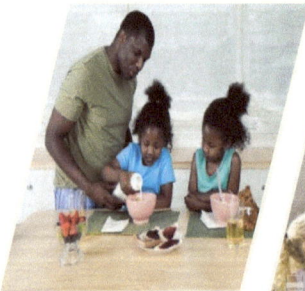

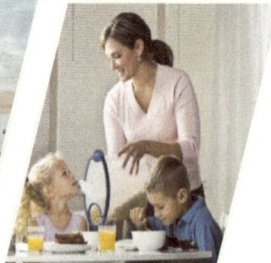

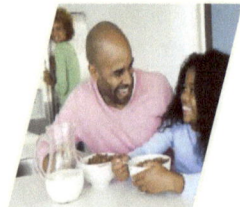

Billie Jean King

Kid Friendly Foods

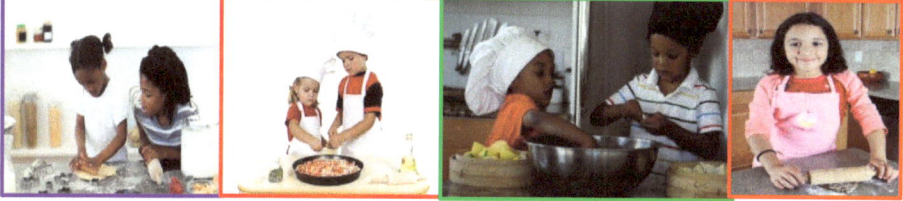

Concerning these recipes, they're designed more to point you toward healthier eating choices and options. When I began preparing some of these dishes, I had no recipe for them. I just went into the kitchen and started preparing them the way I thought that they should taste. I was old school taught, you know, "*a little dash of this, and a pinch or two of that.*" So, please grade me on a curve and think out of the box and incorporate your own imagination and cooking experience. After trying them a few times, you'll eventually get it the way that you like it. For these recipes and suggestions, I have kids in mind, but, this will become a family favorite. Everyone loves burgers, cheese burgers and fries. You guessed it, turkey burgers.

Turkey/Cheese Burger

1-lb of ground turkey
1 pk of onion soup mix.

1 pk of whole wheat buns
Cheese slices (optional)

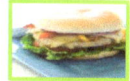

Mix package of onion soup with turkey, blend well. Shape into patties. Cook in skillet, grill, your choice. Let your child or kids mix and shape the patty's, they'll love it, it's better than play dough. Makes about 4 burgers...*yummy!*

- Steak fries- cut in large sections. Spray baking pan with non stick spray. Sprinkle on your choice of seasoning. Place in oven and bake until golden brown. If using frozen French fries, experiment, place on baking pan and bake.

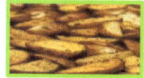

- Yogurt – Graham Cracker Parfait- Using a small or large container, layer the bottom with crumpled graham crackers. Add a layer of your favorite yogurt. Repeat the process until container is filled. Sit in fridge until crackers soften, 1-2 hours. *Yum...Taste like you're eating cheesecake, or add bananas, and you've got a banana pudding. Great for dessert or a snack.*

Let's Get Steppin!

- **Sweet Potato/Yam Fries-** Cut sweet potato or yams in strips. Place on sprayed baking sheet. Sprinkle with cinnamon, to kick up the flavor, sprinkle on a little cayenne pepper. Baked until cooked.

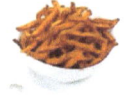

- **Italian Turkey Sausage Pizza**, Boboli makes great whole wheat pizza dough, it includes the sauce. Load dough with pieces of Italian turkey sausage, and your favorite pizza toppings and cheese. Place in oven and bake.

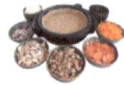

- **Whole Wheat Bagel Pizza Snacks**- slice bagel open, spread on tomato based sauce, sprinkle with sausage and cheese or no sausage, just add cheese and melt in oven or microwave. Makes a great snack.

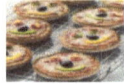

- **Tortilla Chips**- to make homemade tortilla chip, buy a bag of 100% whole wheat pita pocket bread. From the opening of the pocket, use scissors cut open pocket. This will give you to whole round pieces. Fold each in half and cut in the shape of triangles until all are completed. Place on sprayed cooking sheet, sprinkle with your favorite seasons and bake until crisp.

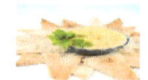

- **Old Fashion Popcorn Snacks**- remember popcorn before the microwave. Some will say, No! Try popping kernels of corn in hot air popper, or from a covered container on the stove. Kids will love to hear the popping sound as they watch the kernels become white and fluffy. This method allows you to control the sodium content without additives.

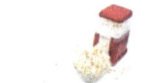

- **Apple Snacks**-Kids love gadgets, using an apple slicer, pear in sections, leave the apples on the slicer and allow the kids to remove it a slice at a time. It's great for dipping into peanut butter, fat free caramel, or having for a snack. (*you can find them for $1.00 at .99 cent and $ stores.*)

63

Billie Jean King

Whole Wheat Pancakes

1cup of 100% whole wheat
¼ teaspoon of salt
½ teaspoon of sugar

1 level teaspoon of baking powder pastry flour

¾ cup of milk or water

Combine ingredients, mix well, spray griddle or skillet with a non stick solution, pour on batter and cook. You can add your choice of fruits, banana, blue berries strawberries, or top with your favorite syrup or fruit.

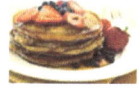

Whole Wheat Waffles -Use the same ingredients as pancakes.

- *Wheat and pastry flour can be costly. Try purchasing it at your local super market on their bulk aisle. Safeway, Nobhill, Raleys and Winco have bulk items.*

Whole Wheat French Toast-

Use 100% sliced whole wheat bread. Eggs, Milk, pinch of salt. Combine ingredients. Soak slices of bread on   both sides and place on cooking surface until golden brown.

I know, you're saying; *"where's the meat."* Remember…for breakfast, we're limited in our choices of healthy meats. Processed turkey sausages have been available in the frozen food section of our grocery stores for some time now. However, they are pre-cooked with high sodium content and other additives; and they lack the title of being referred to as a healthier breakfast meat choice, along with beef bacon. Even kids love having meat as a side dish over cereal and milk, when Mom decides to treat them to toast, eggs, sausages, pancakes and waffles.

Recently I began to experiment with making ground *turkey breakfast sausages*. For years, I'd used it instead of ground beef with pasta dishes; so why not *sausages*. I included spices that I love; you can try your favorites. I'm merely attempting to offer alternatives.

Homemade Turkey Breakfast Sausages

1lb Ground Turkey
Garlic and onion powder
Sage- add to your taste

1 package of onion soup mix
Black Pepper
Cayenne Pepper
(*if you like it spicy*)

Incorporate ingredients the way you'd prepare a meatloaf. Once thoroughly blended, separate into patties or role into sausage links. Cook them in the oven, on a sprayed pan, fry in skillet, or a George Foreman grill.   (**Sodium Free Diet:** Omit the onion soup mix, substitute with spices.)

Tip: *Make a batch of sausage patties & links. They freeze well.*
Note: *Always check the ingredients for parts of turkey that's included.*

Let's Get Steppin!

Homemade Turkey Sausage Omelet

Eggs   diced potatoes
Diced homemade turkey sausage   cheese
Onions/ white or green   bits of garlic

Before mixing egg batter, dice a small white or russet potato. Cook in microwave or boil until soft. Prepare egg batter, Place in skillet. When eggs become firm, add remainder of ingredients including potatoes. Save some cheese for topping. No additional salt needed, cheese and sausage will add flavor. You can fold omelet in half, or leave open faced and top with cheese...Yum!

Egg and Homemade Turkey Sausage Bagel

1 multi grain bagel or whole wheat bagel
1 egg
Slice bagel, heat in toaster, or microwave, after breaking and seasoning egg, place   in a container the size of your bagel. The bottom of a cup or bowl works well. Cook until done, generally one minute or less. Place cooked egg and sausage patty onto bagel. Eat plain or add your favorite jam, jelly, or whatever.

Egg Bagel: Prepare the same way, excluding sausage.(Safeway bakery makes great multi grain bagels)

Yogurt Parfait: 1 cup of yogurt, **top** with granola or any whole grain cereal. Your choice of fruit, slices of bananas, strawberries, or blue berries,

Oatmeal: topped with cinnamon, raisins, walnuts, blue berries.
(*Steel Oats contains more fiber.*)

Billie Jean King

Manufacturers- Alternative Food Selections-Tips:

You've heard of the expression, *"where there is a will, there is a way."* It holds true for food as well. Thank God for the manufacturers that have increased their product line to include wheat, whole grain and brown rice. Boxed pasta or rice entree can be exchanged with brown rice or whole grain pasta of your choosing. Keep in mind, the flavor that we love is in the contents of the packet of seasoning that's included, not the pasta. Remember, Ground Turkey works great with these boxed entrees also.

Ramen and Noodles in a cup:

Noodles N a Cup　　*Ramen Noodles*　　*Wheat Pasta*

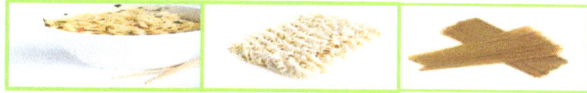

I have yet to find any ramen or noodles in a cup in whole grain, but all is not loss, I make substitutions that provide me with a level of satisfaction. By substituting the ramen or noodles in a cup with whole grain spaghetti and using the manufacturer's packet of seasoning, I still enjoy the delicious flavor that I've grown to love. If you're watching your sodium intake, you might consider using half the packet of seasoning. Both are loaded with sodium.

Boxed Entrée's:

Brown Rice　　*Assorted Wheat Pasta*　　*Ground Turkey*

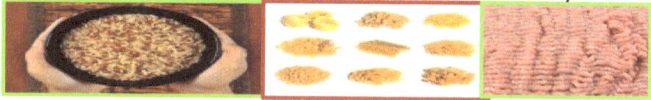

We all love our hamburger helper dishes; check your grocery aisle, you'll find several whole grain selections. Rice A Roni, have a brown rice option, along with Uncle Ben, Success Rice, and Zatarian to highlight a few. Love Mac & Cheese, with kids in mind, Kraft have a box with individual packets of whole grain mac & cheese.

Boxed pasta or rice entree can be exchanged with brown rice or whole wheat pasta of your choosing. Keep in mind, the flavor that we love is in the contents of the packet of seasoning that's included, *not the pasta.* Remember, Ground Turkey works great with these boxed entrees also. Do not be surprised when you go to your favorite grocery store and can't find the above items. Grocery stores stock foods that are in demand by their shoppers. If you're persistent in your request, they will stock it.

Burrito:

Burrito　　*Wheat Tortilla Brown Rice*　　*Black Beams Ground Turkey*

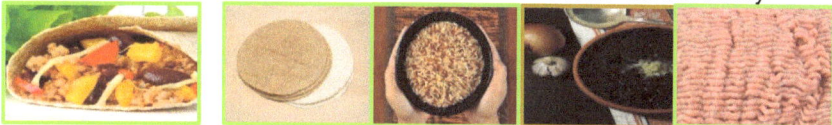

Who said a burrito can't be healthy? Black beans and wheat flour tortilla offer a natural source of fiber over refried beans. Black beans are high in protein and antioxidant.

66

Let's Get Steppin!

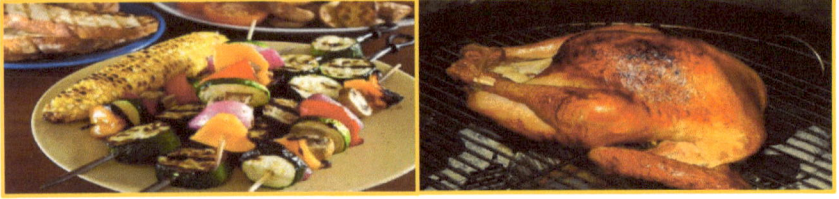

Summer is a great time for grilling. For some reason, smoked meat is so tasty, and it doesn't require a lot of seasoning. Depending on your area, the summer months can get pretty heated, and who wants to be stuck in a hot kitchen every day. Try smoking a turkey, not frying it. You do not need a smoker; any grill with a cover will work.

- Season the turkey with your choice of spices. Wrap it in foil and place on the grill with cover down. The idea is to smoke it. Adding wood chips gives it a robust smoked flavor. Smoke it slowly, it doesn't require constant attention.
- If you're pressed for time and it has smoked for at least two hours; remove and place in oven with foil until fully cooked. The results will be great. You'll have a tender smoked tasting turkey.
- While the coals are still hot. Make some turkey kabobs. Your kids will love making and eating them.
- Use the breast of the turkey for the kabobs. Cut in large squares, add your favorite veggies, cut up red potatoes, sliced zucchini, mushrooms, and place on a stick, season and grill. *Remember, the whole idea is to give Mom a break from the stove while eating healthy. I recall going about three days without cooking.*

Sub Turkey Sandwich: Whole wheat hoagie rolls. Pile   on sliced or diced turkey, peppers, onions, tomatoes, pickles, cucumbers, olives. Can't find the hoagie rolls, use whole wheat sliced bread, or whole wheat hamburger buns. This is great for lunch or dinner.

Turkey Salad: Using your favorite part of the turkey, cut in small pieces. Adding miracle whip, or mayo, throw in some chopped onions, white or green, bell pepper, sweet pickles or relish and, paprika.. Mix well, have a turkey salad sandwich or place on opened faced crackers.

Garden Salad: Over a bed of lettuce or spinach. Toss on some diced turkey breast or any part of the turkey, dried cranberries, boiled eggs, salad dressing, tomatoes and cucumbers. A scoop of turkey salad over lettuce or spinach works too.

Hot meal- With dark meat portions, slice and heat to serve with brown rice or mashed potatoes and your favorite veggies or salad. Come thanksgiving, you'll want more.

Ground Beef Favorites...
Substituted With Ground Turkey

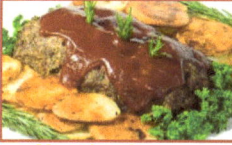 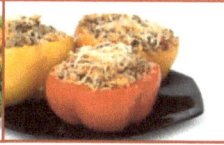 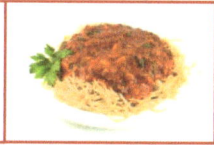 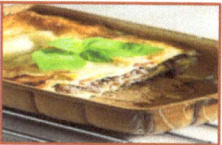

Meat Loaf   Stuffed Bell Peppers   Spaghetti   Lasagna

For generations, ground beef has been an all time favorite staple to take to potlucks and special events. Ground turkey is on the rise to being the up-and-coming substitute for ground beef dishes. Below is a list of foods that works just as great with ground turkey.

Lasagna: Use whole grain wide noodle. To reduce fat and dairy content, replace ricotta cheese with cottage cheese. Using ground turkey, prepare as you would using ground beef. Complete with your favorite ingredients.

Pasta Dishes: With whole grain pasta's such as, spaghetti, rigatoni, penne, and mostacholi, using your favorite seasoning, prepare your meat sauce as you would with ground beef.

Meat Loaf: Incorporate your favorite meat loaf seasoning and spices with a pound or two of ground turkey meat.

Stuffed Bell Peppers: Prepare the meat as you would for a meat sauce, stuff into a pepper and bake until meat and peppers are done.

IN the previous pages I illustrated images of foods that if eaten in **excess** will eventually lead to obesity and the related diseases. The following pages will depict illustrations of foods that will promote good health if we incorporate them into our daily diet.

Let's Get Steppin!

FOODS HIGH IN FIBER- GRAINS-ANTIOXIDANTS-BETA CAROTENE

Cereal	Bran Muffin	Wheat Bread	Beans

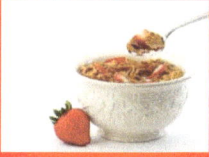 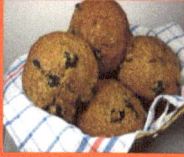 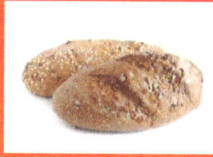 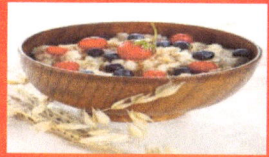

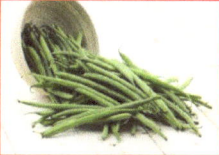 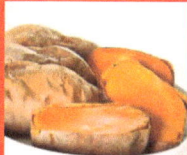 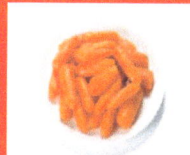 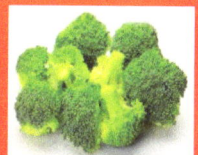

Collard Greens	Corn	Spinach	

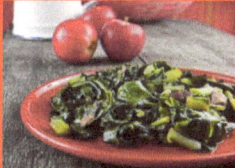 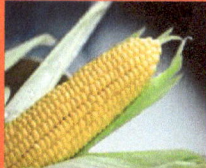 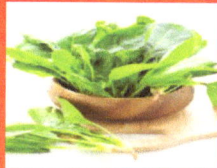 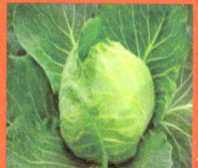

Lentils	Squash	Tomatoes	Swiss Chard

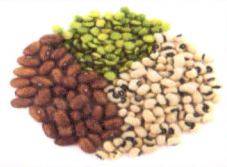 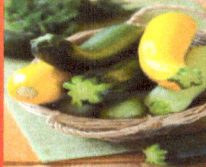 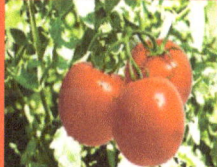 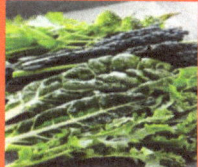

Cucumbers	Avocados	Bok Choy

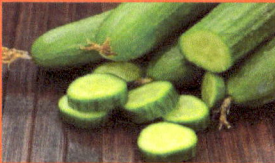 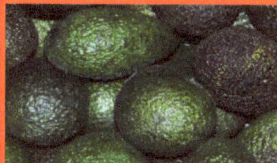 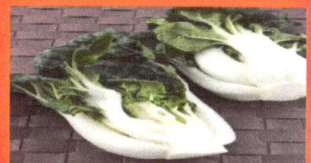

Granola Bars	Mixed Nuts-Raisins	Almonds

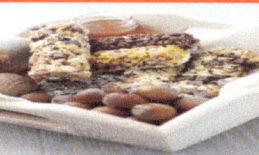 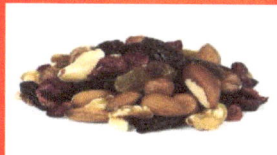 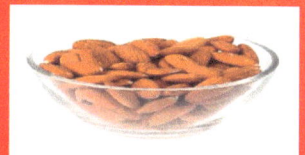

Healthy Fruit Snacks
Rich In Vitimins - Antioxidants

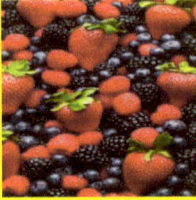

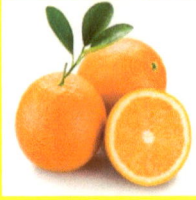

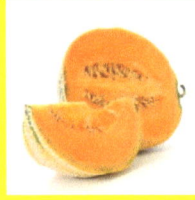

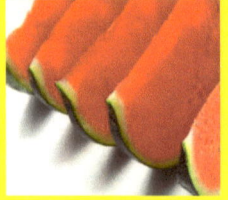

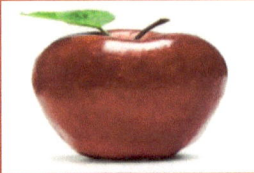

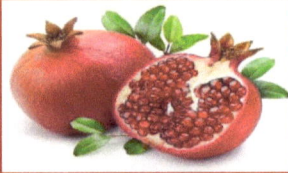

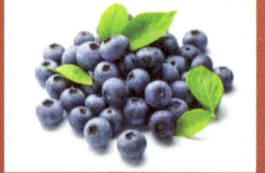

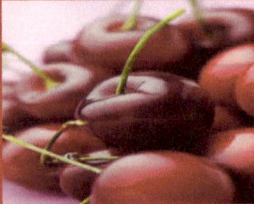

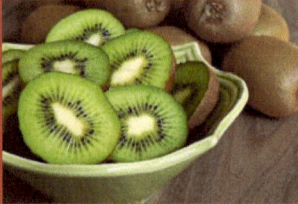

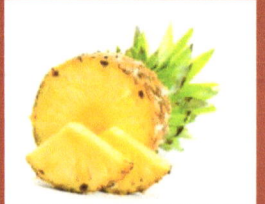

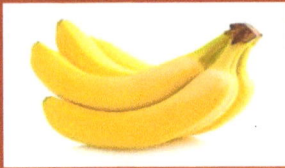

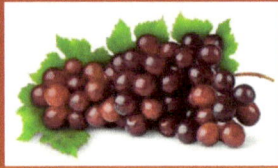

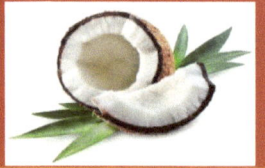

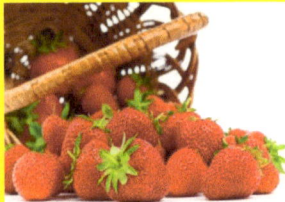

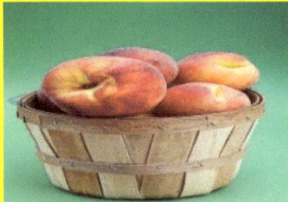

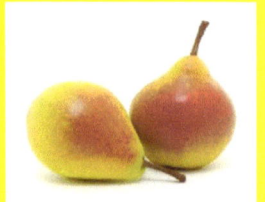

FOODS RICH IN PROTIEN-OMGA 3

Salmon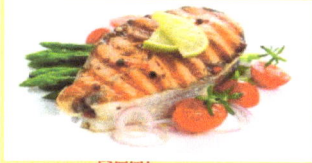

Grilled Tuna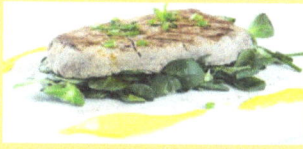

Canned Tuna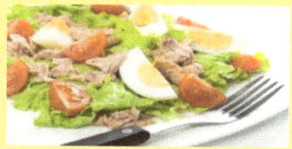

Beef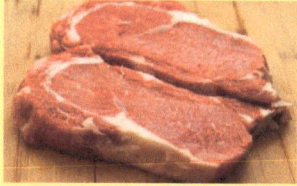

Pork Chops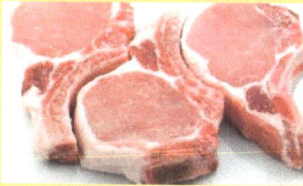

Whole Milk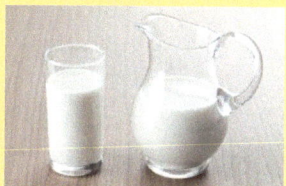

Assorted Cheeses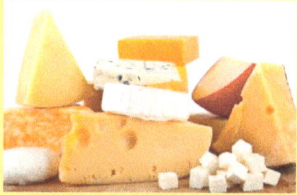

Chicken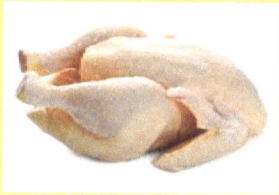

Almonds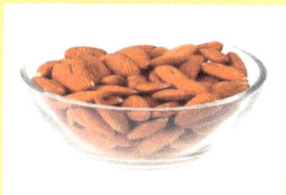

Black Beans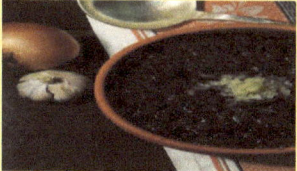

Peanut Butter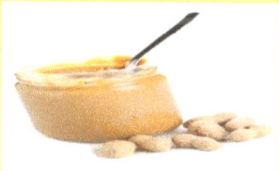

Eggs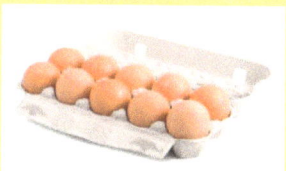

Cottage Cheese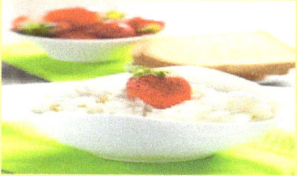

Yogurt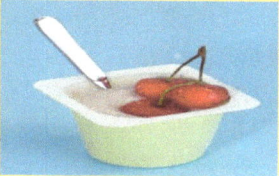

Flax Seeds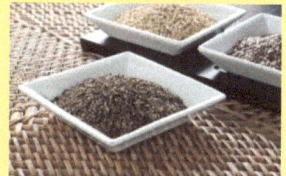

Set Back-Aunt Diagnosed with Alzheimer's Disease

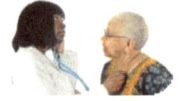

Definition: Alzheimer's disease: A progressive neurologic disease of the brain that leads to the irreversible loss of neurons and dementia. The clinical hallmarks of Alzheimer's disease are progressive impairment in memory, judgment, decision making, and orientation to physical surroundings, and language. *(MedicineNet.com)*

This is a disease that's soaring among the elderly. However, recent studies have given us a reason for hope. Although the disease is associated with the neurological section of a person's brain, the effects impacts and encroaches upon the family and the caregiver, which is generally a spouse or family member.

June of 2010, my 85 year old aunt was diagnosed with the Alzheimer's disease. If you noticed, a major portion of my book was written in the present tense as events were unfolding in 2009 and 2010. After this revelation, it did not afford me the time or the mindset to continue writing.

After enduring the challenges presented as being the only caregiver; I can testify to the helplessness, and frustration that can lead to stress and depression. I recall one overwhelming evening in particular after leaving her home. I consciously went to the store, purchased a half of gallon of chocolate mint ice cream, and a bag of chocolate cookies. After scooping up a generous portion of ice cream, I covered it with whole and crumbled cookies. If that wasn't enough, I had the *audacity* to get in bed and eat it while watching TV. I can't remember what I was watching; I was too busy nursing my frustrations. I ate it so fast; I didn't allow myself the time to contemplate what I was doing.

At that moment, it tasted so good; it gave me the comfort that I was so desperately seeking. As I walked to the sink to put away the bowl and spoon, I finally took ownership of what had transpired. With God as my only witness, I placed the remainder of the container of ice cream into the sink and filled it with water. I placed the remaining two rows of cookies in the water on top of the ice cream. From previous experience I knew that when I returned later that I would be sickened by an image of foamy ice cream and expanded soggy cookies. It would serve as a good aversion therapy treatment for future enticements.

Let's Get Steppin!

Yes, I was able to get a handle on the situation and prevent further damage, but it proved how stress from the circumstances in life can cause us to give in to the temptation of *Gluttony.* Remember earlier I mentioned how I only bring home a slice of cake and a 2 oz carton of ice cream to satisfy the craving,…I feel that some clarification is in order.

Possessing the will power to toss the ice cream and cookies came from *years of cultivating that mind set.* I don't want you to think that you can go out and buy a large quantity of your favorite foods and fool yourself into thinking that you can easily toss it after you've gotten your fix. Do not be deceived…trust me, you'll end up eating all of it before the day or night is over. And if the calories exceeds 3500 hundred; you will have succeeded in rewarding yourself with an *extra pound.* After I took ownership of what I'd done; in spite of my frustrated state of mind, I knew that it was time to toss the *goodies.*

I had a conversation with a friend about this situation a month ago. We were discussing how we handle the excess of food that's been brought into the home after we know that we've had our limit. She shared how her husband will throw it away after he's satisfied his craving. I enthusiastically responded, "*me too.*" She went on to say that she had not arrived at that level of will power… yet! Trust me; you will be flirting with a temptation you will not be able to resist.

In September of 2010, Good Morning America aired a segment on the Alzheimer's disease; Maria Shriver was the featured guest. Maria introduced her "*A Woman's Nation Takes on Alzheimer's.* According to Maria, 65% of the epidemic is held by women. Since the large percentages of caregivers are women, the risk to acquire it is greater. From research they've keyed in on the fact that the onset of the disease may occur in women as early as in their 40's and 50's, during menopause. It's proclaimed as being a twenty year disease in the making. You may be thinking, "*why is she sharing this, it has nothing to do with walking, kids, or obesity.*" As stated by Maria, **Type II Diabetics, Obesity and Depression** are known contributors to developing the disease.

After learning of this information; I felt compelled to highlight its association with Obesity and Type II Diabetes. For more information on Maria's report, and to see the video, visit www.ABC.COM/GMAC

In late September of 2010, after securing a comfortable facility for my aunt, I was able to resume my writing. Consistent to three of the known contributors to the disease, my aunt bore all three.

Final Thoughts . . .

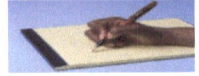

The word diet in association to losing weight has become synonymous to the meaning of *deprivation.* Denial is one of the primary reasons why we're never able to stay on a *reducing diet* long enough to achieve the results that it proclaims. It's unfortunate, but a large number of *us* have placed our health in such jeopardy by satisfying our robust appetites, until *we have no recourse now but to submit to some level of depravity.* That is, if we want to live healthy and productive lives, for some, just live. Ideally, a life that is free of taking high blood pressure, high cholesterol, diabetes, and heart medications. These medications serve only as a temporary "crutch" for a few decades to suppress the foreseeable health effects from the consequences of our over indulgence. They only provide us with a *false sense* of comfort while we enjoy excessive food pleasures thinking that we're beating the odds. Histories of poor health conditions support the fact that we are not beating the odds.

My aim was to share some of the alterative measures that I've incorporated into my daily living; measures that produced a lifestyle of making better choices. If I had to choose three words to convey my message; they would be *balance, sacrifice and movement.* Balance would include consuming all five food groups daily, carbohydrates, (whole grains) vegetables, fruits, fat, and diary; and not limiting it to carb's and fats. Sacrifice is denying or limiting the intake of our favorite carb's and fats in a given time period. Movement simply means to get active doing something.

If the familiar old adage of, "*if it's worth having, it's worth working hard to get it"* is true; then, how valuable is our health? We place great value on acquiring money, and our pet material possessions; yet, without good health, we become limited in acquiring them. The most devastating scenario is to gain it all and then to be denied the pleasure of enjoying it due to self inflicted poor health from over indulgence. Without conscious, we've allowed our eyes, and our taste buds to dictate the amount of food that we consume. In all truthfulness, *we eat primarily because of how good food tastes to us.* When we're on our second and third helping of food; the hunger has long been satisfied. How many times have you said, *"Hmm..?I'm eating now because it's good!* Amen…!

The type of foods that I've mentioned and listed are not foods that I came up with on my own; aside from my recipes, they are food groups that we hear every day from public service announcements, commercials, dieticians , nutritionist, health based talk shows, and our doctors.

Let's Get Steppin!

The food selections are not advocating weight loss, but if eaten in moderation and limited portions; you can maintain your weight if that's your goal. On the other hand, employing the same principles and including movement such as walking, exercising, and other physical activities; you can certainly lose the weight. For some of you, my story and information will serve only as affirmation, to some, as preventive measures, and that's a blessing. But, I'm certain that some of you or each of you will have a family member or a close friend that would benefit from some alternative food choices and the need to incorporate some extracurricular activity into your daily living.

It would be remiss of me if I didn't share the most crucial aspect of what keeps me inspired. Pedometer walking, the lifestyle change in eating habits are definitely contributing factors; but there was an internal change and determination that existed as well.

In 2005, I realized that I possessed the ability to exhort and encourage through my writing and speaking abilities. It's also when I discovered my God given purpose. At each awaking day, my inspiration was magnified as I attempted to complete my desired dreams and goals. My yearning to take better care of my body increased immensely; which accelerated and propelled my walking and the desire to make a change in my eating behavior and food selections.

Imagine this, the moment that you can see that there's light at the end of the tunnel; all sorts of possibilities are open. Suddenly, a new you will emerge, with a new and purposed minded agenda. Your days are spent planning and strategizing how you're going to pursue and accomplish this newly found passion. You may even experience a few sleepless nights; but it won't be from worry. Metaphorically speaking, it's reminiscent of a new found love, remember the excitement.

No longer will you be defined by your birth or occupation *identity* alone; but, you'll have definition that's characterized by your God given abilities, talents and gifts. *I strongly believe, until I uncovered my purpose for being here; I would've continued to mask my obstacles, setbacks and disappointments in life with excessive food consumption.* As with anything or people that we love, we take care of them. Especially our cars, in order to get the maximum performance from our cars; we only put into it the manufactures recommended type of fuel and oil. To perform at our maximum potential for our new found purpose and aspirations, we're going to need a *healthy body* to succeed.

I can imagine by now you're mumbling, "*I'm too old for change.*" From one to another, don't be afraid to become a "*late bloomer.*" Experience has it rewards and privileges. You may be saying, "*I have no clue of why I'm here.*" If you have no idea , try compiling a "*bucket list.*" You just might be surprised that something that you've always wanted to do may be your *purpose.*

Billie Jean King

Until you discover that "*thing*" that makes you excited to get out of bed; and then hate it when it's time for you to go back to bed; try devoting each day toward finding it. Experts advocate that, *that thing which we do so well, without effort or thought daily, is generally our gift.* I have to confess that was the case for me. I always loved to write. If confrontation was in order, or I needed to express or share my emotions with a significant other or my daughter; writing was always my choice of communication. Validation was in order when one recipient responded, *"I always enjoy reading your letters, and everything flows so smoothly."* My daughter would often seek my opinions and suggestions in writing her college term papers. These comments were later recognized as confirmation. I shared that for you to be *mindful of compliments and praises that you may get from your inner circle of individuals or family members on things that you've done.*

As a final point, our children… which was my inspiration for writing this book. Until we as parents, grandparents, aunts, and uncles can reconcile what's eating us; discover our purpose for this life; place our dreams and inspirations over eating; our kids will be encumbered to repeat the "curse" of Obesity. It will be natural a progression for them to continue to coexist in the environment of food choices that we've created for them. It's well documented that we become our surroundings, from one… generation to the… other.

Since the bible days, testimonies have served as a witness to various accounts and events. No commercial or ad can replace the impact of a personal testimony, it's why you'll find them on numerous business websites advocating for that particular product or service that they've used. From the pages of this book, I've attempted to share my testimony of how walking with the aid of the pedometer motivated and propelled me toward cultivating a lifestyle of consistent walking.

After realizing the positive role that walking carried on the impact of warding off the known diseases associated with obesity; it's no longer viewed as a chore. My last cholesterol check produced me a total number of 140, blood pressure 128/78, and blood sugar of 90. Clinically speaking, whether I'm categorized as being fat, obese, or unhealthy; I consider it a privilege and a blessing to maintain the stamina and the motivation to walk for an hour or more daily. I attribute my energy level to the food choices that I make daily. As stated in my introduction, I remain in the struggle with you. So…Let's Get Steppin!

With Heartfelt Sincerity,

Billie Jean King

www.billiejeankingatlast.com

78

"Let's Get Steppin", America.. Saving…the Next Generation.

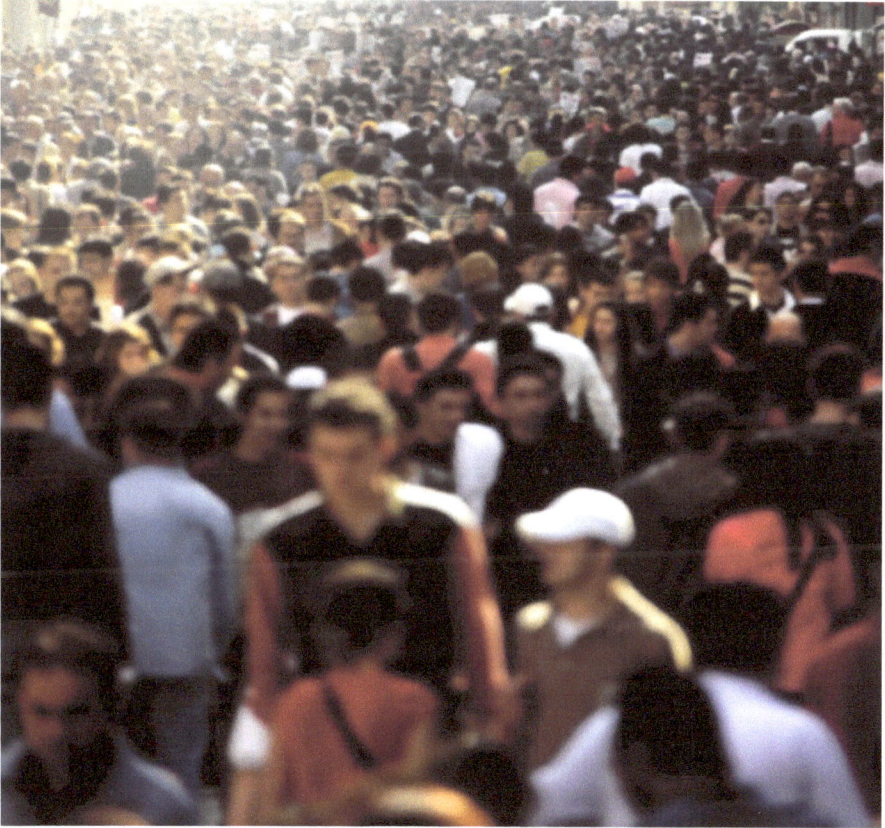

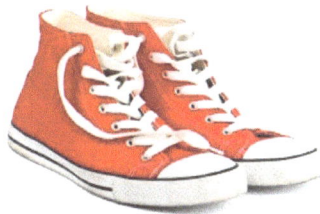

GLOSSARY

(Terms associated with obesity and the related diseases.)

Antioxidants: are chemicals that can protect against damage to cells induced by free radicals and other oxidative processes. Antioxidants are found in a variety of foods, especially in brightly colored fruits and vegetables. Vitamins, such as vitamins E and C, are also considered antioxidants.

Average Activity Levels Monitored by Pedometer:

Blood Glucose: the main sugar that the body makes from the food in the diet. Glucose is carried through the bloodstream to provide energy to all cells in the body cells cannot use glucose without the help of insulin.

Blood Pressure: the blood pressure is the pressure of the blood within the arteries. It is produced primarily by the contraction of the heart of the heart muscle. Its measurement is recorded by two numbers. The first (systolic pressure) is measured after the heart contracts and lowest. A blood pressure cuff is used to measure the pressure. Elevation of blood pressure is called "hypertension".

Calorie: is a measure of energy expenditure. The calories referred to in diet and exercises are kilocalories (kcal) – 1000 of the calories referred to in science labs for measuring chemical reactions. A proud of fat equals 3500 calories.

Carbohydrates: mainly sugars and starches, together constituting one of the here principle types of nutrients used as energy sources (calories) by the body. There are two types of Carb's.

- Simple Carb's commonly known as " bad carb's)
  Table Sugar-Cakes, Biscuits, Soft Drinks, Candy
  White Rice and Pasta.
- Complex Carb's are referred to as "good carb's."
  Bran, Wheat, Whole Breads, Oatmeal, Brown Rice, Wholegrain Pasta, Wholegrain Cereals, Fibers, Beans, lentils.

Cholesterol: is a chemical compound that is naturally produced by the body and is a combination of lipid (fat) and steroid. Cholesterol is a building block for cell membranes and for hormones like estrogen and testosterone.

About 80% of the body's cholesterol is produced by the liver, while the rest comes from our diet. Dietary cholesterol comes mainly from meat, poultry, fish and dairy products.

Let's Get Steppin!

Congestive Heart Failure: inability of the heart to keep up with the demands on it, and specifically, failure of the heart to pump blood with normal efficiency. When this occurs, the heart is unable to provide adequate blood flow to other organs such as the brain, liver and kidneys.

Diet: the sum total of your daily food intake.

Diabetes Type I: an autoimmune disease that occurs when T cells attack and decimate the beta cells in the pancreas that are needed to produce insulin, so that the pancreas makes too little insulin (or no insulin). Without the capacity to make adequate amounts of insulin, the body is not (ketoacids) build up in the body. There is a genetic predisposition to Type I Diabetes. This disease tends to occur in childhood, adolescence or early adulthood (before age 30) but it may have its clinical onset at any age.

Diabetes Type II: In Type II Diabetes, the beta cells produce insulin but cells throughout the body do not respond normally to it. Nevertheless, insulin also may be used in type II diabetes to help overcome the resistance of cells to insulin.

Exercise/Movement: To set in action; to cause to act, move, or make exertion, to in action habitually or repeatedly.

Fiber: is defined as a material made by plants that is not digested by the human gastrointestinal tract. Fiber is one of the mainstays in the treat of constipation. Foods that's high in fiber.

- Broccoli, spinach, grains, brown rice, whole wheat breads, air popped corn, oat bran, collard, cabbage greens, and yams.

Heart Attack: the death of heart muscle due to the loss of blood supply. The loss of blood supply is usually caused by a complete blockage of a coronary artery, one of the arteries that supplied blood to the heart muscle. Death of the heart muscle, in turn, causes chest pain and electrical instability of the heart muscle tissue.

Heart Disease: any disorder that affects the heart. Sometimes the term "heart disease" is used narrowly and incorrectly as a synonym for coronary artery disease.

High Fructose Corn Syrup: is a sweetener made from corn and can be found in numerous foods and beverages on grocery store shelves in the United States.

High Blood Pressure: also known as hypertension, high blood pressure exceeding 140 over 90 mmHg-a systolic pressure above 140 with a diastolic pressure above 90. (*Recent studies have revised these numbers.)*
Hydrogenated Vegetables Oils: produces Tran's fat. Manufacturers add androgen to the vegetable oil. Hydrogenation increases the shelf life and flavor stability of foods containing these fats.

Insulin: A natural hormone made by the pancreas that controls the level of the sugar glucose in the blood. Insulin permits cells to use glucose for energy. Cells cannot utilize glucose without insulin.

Kidney: One of a pair of organs located in the right and left side of the abdomen which clear "poisons" from the blood, regulate acid concentration and maintain water balance in the body

Obesity: the definition of obesity varies depending on what one reads, but in general, it is a chronic condition defined by an excess amount of body fat, well above one's normal weight.

Renal Kidney: Renal failure is a condition where the kidneys lose their normal functionality, which may be due to various factors including infections, auto immune diseases, diabetes and other endocrine disorders, such as cancer.

Toxic Chemicals: it usually occurs at the terminal stages of the disease process. Once renal failure occurs, it requires immediate management and even then prognosis is often not good unless transplantation is done.

Sedentary Life Style: A sedentary lifestyle is defined as engaging in no leisure-time physical activity (exercises, sports, physically active hobbies.)

Sleep Apnea: is a disorder characterized by a reduction or pause of breathing (airflow) during sleep. It is common among adults but rare among children. An apnea is a period of time during which breathing stops or is markedly reduced. In simplified terms, an apnea occurs when a person stops breathing for 10 seconds or more.

Stroke: the sudden death of some brain cells due to a lack of oxygen when the blood flow to the heart is impaired by blockage or rupture of an artery to the brain.
A stroke is also called a cerebrovascular accident or, for short, a CVA

Let's Get Steppin!

Trans Fat: Unlike other fats, the majority of Tran's fat is formed when food manufacturers turn liquid oils into solid fats like shortening and hard margarine. Small amounts of Trans fat is found naturally, primarily in some animal based foods. Trans fat, saturated fat and dietary cholesterol, raises the LDL (or "bad") cholesterol that increases your risk for CHD. (Coronary heart disease.)

Reference: MedicineNet.com

What's a What Whole Grain? A whole grain contains all three of the grain kernel:

- Bran: The outer shell that provides fiber, B vitamins and trace minerals.
- Endosperm: The middle part that supplies carbohydrates and protein.
- Germ: The inner part that provides antioxidants, vitamin E and B vitamins.

Whole Grain, is it a food? Is it an ingredient?

A whole grain can be food itself or an ingredient in other foods. For instance: brown rice, popcorn and oatmeal are whole grain foods that often are simply prepared and eaten.

- Whole wheat, whole cornmeal and whole rye are whole grains often used as ingredients in other foods such as bread, crackers and pasta.

Food label lingo: Statements about whole grains on food labels can mean very different things.

- 100% whole grain. All the grain in the product is whole grain.
- Whole-grain food. The product contains at least 51% whole grain by weight.
- Gram amounts, some packages tell you how many grams of whole grains a serving contains. *The 2005 Dietary Guidelines for Americans recommend eating at least three one-ounce equivalents (totaling 48 grams) of whole grains daily for good health.*

Reference: The report of Dietary Guidelines Advisory Committee on Dietary Guidelines for Americans, 2005. Part D Science Base, Section 6: Selected Foods Groups; Fiber and the observed protective effect of whole grain.

Billie Jean King

HELPFUL RESOURCES

Office of the Surgeon General
www.surgeongeneral.gov/

U.S. Dept of Health & Human
Services, ASPE.hhs.gov

American Diabetics Ass.
www.diabetes.org

www.MedicineNet.com

FDA-U.S. Food & Drug Admin
www.fda.gov/

www.Kelloggsnutrition.com

CDC-Center for Disease Control
www.cdc.org

www.helpwithcooking.com

Maria Shriver "A Woman's Nation
Takes on Alzheimer's."
ABC.Com/GMAC

www.sportline.com

Dr. Emit Oz
www.sharecare.com

Dr. Doris Day
www.sharecare.com

Let's Get Steppin!

TRACK YOUR STEPS

Date	Steps Taken During School or Work	Duration	Steps Taken After School or Work	Total For The Day

Billie Jean King

NOTES

86

Let's Get Steppin!

Acknowledgements

Always… giving thanks to God!

Thanks Jordyn! For your brilliant off the cuff expression that later became the title for my book. After you'd completed reading the chapter on you; you leaned back in your chair, followed by a brief sigh…showing an expression of approval; you remarked, "Well…*Let's Get Steppin*! It's far better than the one I had chosen. Thanks!

Thanks DC! Thank you for periodically calling to inquire about the progress of my book and project. It always prompted me to get back on track after I'd encountered setbacks or obstacles. Your resiliency, dedication and commitment toward your projects in your quest for entrepreneurship is addicting and motivating. Thanks a bunch for the patent information and your clever suggestion for my chains.

Thank You! Thank You! Microsoft. Thanks to the technical department team of Perpena, Anishita, Mohammed, and Abdu in India. Thank you for the combined time of **six hours** that you devoted to re-formatting my entire manuscript when my Word software went crazy. You were *Fantastic!*

Thanks Tom! Thank you for your assistance in getting my manuscript in PDF format and compliant ready for print. You were a life saver! Word Mill Publishing & Design. www.wordpr.com

"At Last" ...... *Billie Jean King*

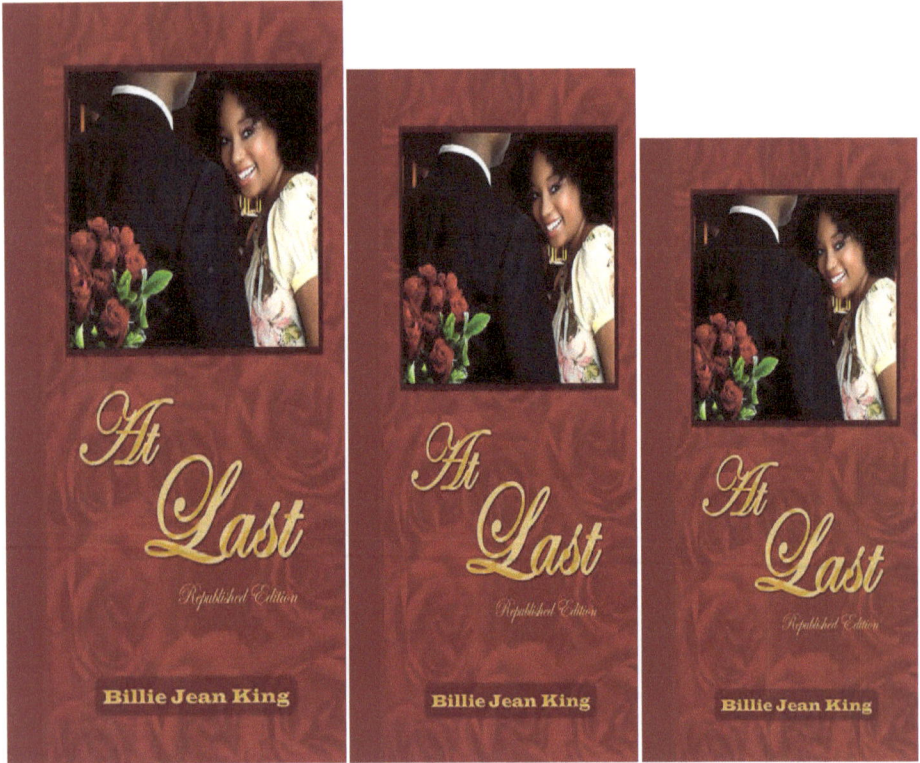

In a Novel that reaffirms the power of *Sisterhood*, Billie Jean King's "At Last" presents a refreshing look at a *bond* between three women of different age groups. When a relationship of sisterhood, friendship, and mentorship is formed; Barbara, Karen and Kim discover that relationship issues faced by singles have no *respect to age*. Being celibate and God fearing women; they've grown weary in their wait for their husbands. In the approaching New Millennium they go on a quest to find their mates; *interracial dating* and *younger men* will be a consideration. A love story unveils as King skillfully illustrates the combination of three women in their new found relationships.

To learn more about this book or to book speaking engagements contact the following.

www.billiejeankingatlast.com atlastbillieking@aol.com

Let's Get Steppin!

Billie Jean King

www.ingramcontent.com/pod-product-compliance
Lightning Source LLC
Chambersburg PA
CBHW041303290326
41931CB00032B/2